ALL SKY, MIRROR OCEAN

ALL SKY

BRAD NECYK

MIRROR

A HEALING MANIFESTO

OCEAN

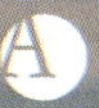

UNIVERSITY *of* ALBERTA PRESS

Published by

University of Alberta Press
1–16 Rutherford Library South
11204 89 Avenue NW
Edmonton, Alberta, Canada T6G 2J4
amiskwaciwâskahikan | Treaty 6 |
Métis Territory
uap.ualberta.ca | uapress@ualberta.ca

LIBRARY AND ARCHIVES CANADA
CATALOGUING IN PUBLICATION

Title: All sky, mirror ocean : a healing manifesto / Brad Necyk.
Names: Necyk, Brad, author, artist.
Description: Includes bibliographical references.
Identifiers: Canadiana (print) 2023022718X | Canadiana (ebook) 20230227228 | ISBN 9781772126778 (softcover) | ISBN 9781772127188 (EPUB) | ISBN 9781772127195 (PDF)
Subjects: LCSH: Necyk, Brad—Mental health. | LCSH: Art and mental illness. | LCSH: Mental healing.
Classification: LCC N71.5 .N43 2024 | DDC 701/.15—dc23

First edition, first printing, 2024.
First printed and bound in Canada by Friesens, Altona, Manitoba.
Copyediting and proofreading by Joanne Muzak.

University of Alberta Press gratefully acknowledges the support received for its publishing program from the Government of Canada, the Canada Council for the Arts, and the Government of Alberta through the Alberta Media Fund.

Canada

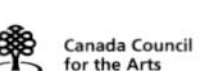

Alberta
Government

for ~~*you*~~
and
~~*me*~~

CONTENTS

ALTERNATIVE TABLE OF CONTENTS

Visionary Art

FOREWORD

There Is a Way through the Heart...And/Or, How to Read This Book

NATALIE LOVELESS

> *The process of conducting this research, creating the art, and writing this book has been the most healing period in my life. This is a healing manifesto.*
>
> —*BRAD NECYK, All Sky, Mirror Ocean*

I write this foreword from an airplane moving from one conflict zone to another, both in desperate need of healing. I write with the weight of histories of genocide practiced in those lands we now call Israel and those we call Canada. I write from the midst of many memories of the heart. These memories inflect my reflection on the book you currently hold in your hands.

Weaving elegantly—and *alchemically*—through anecdote, memory, vignette, and story, Brad's *All Sky, Mirror Ocean* models research-creation at its aesthetic and political best.[1] A journey through bipolar (dis)order, family life, and parenting...climate change, social justice, and medical humanities research...critical disability studies, mad studies, studies in psychiatry and neuroscience...literature, philosophy, and theory...it is a joy to read, and a joy to succumb to the writing's rhythms and flows. Deeply somatic, each page transforms *hurt* (individual, shared, local, global) into *heart*.

Brad writes as an artist and a visionary. From this place, he works to create new spaces for research-creation at the intersection of art and social and ecological justice. Based on years of fieldwork, site visits, ethics permissions, and notes, *All Sky, Mirror Ocean* works at the level of

word

in

relation

to page.

It weaves fragments, snippets, and aphorisms. The rhythms of the shapes on the page in-form our reading. Diaristic excavation of intergenerational family narratives, trauma, loves, joys, and cares meet decolonial-feminist, mad studies, and research-creation perspectives. Together these guide the way.

Indeed, to have the *ears to hear* and receive what *All Sky, Mirror Ocean* offers requires giving oneself over to these word-images and their pacing. It requires wallowing and allowing yourself the

time

to

read.

To read word by word, allowing each to build on the other to create a syncopated interwoven world, dense with allusion, memory, plea, and insight.

Nothing of this text is from without. It is all from within. All worked and worked-through, in both the psychoanalytic and artistic senses of these terms. Reading for *content alone* has no place here. The content of the book is made possible by the forms crafted to share knowledge-as-gift: as situated knowledge.

Knowledge in place, with spirit.

As artist-philosopher Erin Manning might say: the text marks *thought in the act.*[2]

As intergenerational Shoa survivor, artist, and psychoanalytic theorist Bracha Ettinger might say: the text requires *a wit(h)nessing.*[3]

As Tahltan artist Peter Morin might say: the text is *a love song.*[4]

As xwélmexw sound studies scholar Dylan Robinson might say: it requires *guest* rather than *hungry* listening.[5]

As Latinx scholar of race, inequalities, and global change Vanessa Machado de Oliveira might say: it renders impossible the consumptive drives that configure modernity and its configuration of knowledges.[6]

Individualistic-extractive modalities are undone, both in the process of the writing itself (its marked indebtedness) and the reading experience of the text (its rhythms and syncopation of form). *All Sky, Mirror Ocean* reminds us that healing is a journey with no end. As with all journeys in life, the destination only pretends to be the point. It lures. But the journey is the real joy. Even when it hurts.

While there will have been many ways for you to read through this text—following the linear sequence of the pages in all of their lyrical flows; following the alternative table of contents to curate moments and thoughts in new directions—my recommendation is that you start with the Notes on Conditions. Read it at the beginning *and* at the end, whichever version of the adventure that you choose. Feel the difference that each journey makes.

And/or: ignore my prescription entirely and follow the breadcrumbs, flipping to the back every time a word feels

| Marked | (you will know it when you see it, maybe)
// quote //
Emphasis ,, delicate ,, lovingly marked
~~other~~ :: lyrical :: or :: out-of-place {{though not always}}

Weave back and forth. Treat the Notes on Conditions as a set of footnotes[7] that continually recur, interrupting and intervening...co-creating with you.

And/or: annotate the text with your own interventions.

~~Me You~~

we
are
all
in
it

...breathe out,

and

Or...

Notes

1. I use Brad's first name, throughout, by way of marking both my and Brad's disinvestment in colonial/hetero-patriarchal academic writerly norms, as well as marking (non-coincidentally) our friendship, regard, and love.
2. *Thought in the Act: Passages in the Ecology of Experience* (Minneapolis: University of Minnesota Press, 2014) is a beautiful excavation and meditation on research-creation written by Erin Manning together with Brian Massumi.
3. See Bracha L. Ettinger, *The Matrixial Borderspace* (Minneapolis: University of Minnesota Press, 2006). In it she offers a feminist rereading of the Lacanian theory of the subject, highlighting the structural phalogocentrism and anthropocentrism of Lacan's model, working *with* and *alongside* Lacan's insights in a way that respectfully reads and contributes to the Lacanian oeuvre, while rerouting some of its tendrils.
4. See my "Love Songs (to End Hetero-patriarchal, Settler-Colonial, Extractivism)" in *A Companion to Contemporary Art in a Global Framework*, ed. Amelia Jones and Jane Chin Davidson (Chichester: Wiley Blackwell, 2023).
5. Put simply, to listen "hungrily" is to listen extractively—to get somewhere or gain something. To listen as a *guest* is to honour sovereign difference, and allow this to guide one's listening (and action), without cascading into an individualist anxiety of being that requires consumptive assimilative logics; in feminist terms, it is to listen for difference, respectfully; in Indigenous terms (in my learning thus far) it is it to honour treaty logics. See Dylan Robinson, *Hungry Listening: Resonant Theory for Indigenous Sound Studies* (Minneapolis: University of Minnesota Press, 2020). On Treaty, see Sharon H. Venne, "Treaties Made in Good Faith," *Canadian Review of Comparative Literature* 34, no. 1 (2007), 3–16; and Dwayne Donald, "From What Does Ethical Relationality Flow? An Indian Act in Three Artifacts," in *The Ecological Heart of Teaching: Radical Tales of Refuge and Renewal for Classrooms and Communities*, ed. Jackie Seidel and David W. Jardine (New York: Peter Lang, 2016), 10–17.
6. See Vanessa Machado de Oliveira, *Hospicing Modernity: Facing Humanity's Wrongs and the Implications for Social Activism* (Berkeley, CA: North Atlantic Books, 2021).
7. Footnote for page 244 of the Note on Conditions: You are right, Brad. I wanted it to, but it didn't.

ACKNOWLEDGEMENTS

This book was co-created. It is based on my life, research, and art, yet every poem, image, or punctuation was made possible by connection with others:
love
    —falling   merging, one
There have been so many people in my life who are written directly in these pages or others in the spacing between each word. My wife, Candace, has a chapter at the end but my brother, Graham, is nestled in the spaces between. There is a play in //figure| |~~ground~~\\, what is visible and what the visible reflects on: contrast [strife].

Candace, Ellie, and Mary : : this is our story. Ellie and Mary, this is who you are from as you breathe the life to find who you are to. Candace, you are my best friend in this life and all the rest. We have gone through the unimaginable together. You and I have seen each other through heaven and hell. But I would do it over and over again as long as it is with you.

Mom, Dad. Everything comes from you.

A large part of this book is based on my doctoral research in the University of Alberta's Department of Psychiatry. Pamela Brett-MacLean, you took a meeting with me on a June day in 2015 and changed my life by listening to my story then asking if I would like to do a PhD with you. What vision you have! You see what others don't. You put more into me than any supervisor and elevated me beyond what I could have imagined. Because of this, I feel at home now with my research practice. You are the greatest teacher I will ever know.

You introduced me to Andy Greenshaw and he said an artist could do excellent work on mental health. Andy, you provided me with so many of the opportunities for fieldwork. But most importantly you gave me confidence to do something not many had thought of doing. Now, years out of my PhD, you still take my calls and provide me guidance. You are an amazing mentor. Your Being is what I want to reflect out into the world.

So many others went on this journey with me ::

Brian Stonehocker, I met you when you wore a coat that was a cross
    between a suit and a straightjacket.
    <<I knew you were a special kind of human.>>

Minn Yoon, I met you and you invited me onto the head and neck cancer
    project and created the conditions for so many beautiful connections
    and artworks
    to || manifest.

Ivan Silver, I still can't believe you responded to my email and brought me to the Centre for Addiction and Mental Health.

| I just hope I can repay others someday the way you changed my life. |

And so many more that were the conditions for so many manifestations:

Natalie Loveless, Diane Conrad, Sophie Soklaridis, Sean Caulfield, Marilène Oliver, Blair Brennan, and Maria Whiteman.

I am thankful for the support from the Canadian Institutes for Health Research, Social Sciences and Humanities Research Council, Alberta Foundation for the Arts, Canada Council for the Arts, Canadian Depression Research and Intervention Network, University of Alberta, and MacEwan University.

The colour printing of this book would not have been possible without the donations and visions of many: Scott Nelson, the Brian Webb Dance Company, Andy Greenshaw, Andy Bulloch, Dick Averns, the Arts & Humanities in Health & Medicine Program at the University of Alberta, and the Mathison Centre for Mental Health Research and Education at the University of Calgary.

//////////////////////////////////// ====== \\

There are four people who co-created this book with me, weaving in at different times, shining, unconcealing, pure Beings: Dan Harvey, Brian Webb, aAron Munson, and Sha LaBare. What I love about research-creation is it isn't so much a field of scholarship as a process to scholarship. And in this process we can reimagine the independent researcher, singular jewel, and step back and take in all the jewels that reflect in that singular jewel, awakening connection and compassion—the net of jewels.

No one creates alone. Everyone is reflecting everyone else: interbeing.

I wrote this book but I am not the sole author because there are other people who are conditions for its manifestation. Just as the sunflower seed did not create the sunflower, nor did I create this book. The sunflower had conditions such as soil, mycelium, sun, air, gardener, cloud, rain, and many more conditions for its manifestation. This book had many conditions.

Dan Harvey, you have been my friend for a decade. For years, every week <<now living in different provinces>>, as best we can, we meet and talk about philosophy, politics, and art. You have been the gardener of many seeds that would become wonderful understandings and artworks. You are my longest-standing collaborator. You critique my writings and artworks and elevate everything {I/we} do. Much of what I create isn't planned, I am just part of the condition from which works manifest. You helped me nurture those conditions,

critiquing, adding advice, sharing images, or just daydreaming

— falling into the world of a work of art —

Brian Webb, you came into my life only a few years ago. You are a gift. I wish we had a lifetime left to collaborate together. Your belief in the power of art is infectious. I have so enjoyed collaborating on our dance together over the past four years. I love falling into dreams with you

down in the primordial sea at the edge of time.

You were the first person I shared this book with outside of Sha and I was so nervous. I had created something I was so unsure of. I had no reference in my practice to know if it was good or pure madness. But you called me and told me it was beautiful << I almost collapsed with those words >> You gave me the confidence in this work that I did not yet have. Over the next nine months you read and reread the book and gave me amazing critiques. I remember your first piece of advice when I would write:

breath in and breathe out

And you said to me :: no one says breathe in *and* breathe out when they are meditating.

They say:: breathe in,
breathe out

It was these simple but powerful pieces of advice you gave me.

Another time you caught me recycling an older piece of writing into the book. Because of that, I wrote the story "For Mom, For Dad," and it was one of the most powerful healing experiences of my life. I could not have done that without you. Sha began this project with me but you helped me finish it. Thank you, friend.

aAron Munson, there is nothing the linear line of words can do to describe your impact on my life. I'll leave this page exactly as you would want it: empty, emptied,   emptiness.

FOR SHA : ON WRITING

Thank you, Sha. You are a radiant jewel, so beautiful
supernova, forging all the materials that will become you and me.

I see you, friend. No one < + > one

I know you took this on for Jeremy. Your beautiful brother, lost to your open heart, slipping in your veins and out down the tear on your cheek. I know how hard it was to hear my story of bipolar and suicide|reflecting Jeremy

< ever since, ever since   Jeremy Jeremy   Jeremy   Jeremy Jeremy   it's in
right place, heart towards   Jeremy Jeremy   Jeremy Jeremy   Jeremy   woke
singing to the soil holding   *Rāma*   Jeremy Jeremy   beautiful   body   right
place   bathing colour in   *Rāma*   Jeremy   Jeremy   soil   holy   trying
to say, never enough for   Jeremy Jeremy   Jeremy Jeremy   holy   ghost
ever since, once december   Jeremy   Jeremy Jeremy Sha   Jeremy Sha   >

You care tremendously for all the unnamed souls in your soil, on the surface of your skin, and all the unkissed, unborn generations to come. You are weaved and knotted throughout this book and within me. I had a burning sensation to share a story, or a series of stories. But it was in the *<Otherworld>* of no form, locked down and down — deep in the abyssal space —between—. These stories were scuffed and no one. I could not write these stories. I tried...I wrote 51,000 words and shared it with you. You said:

write the book in one word, but I needed three:

the visionary artist

now I wonder if : healing ; wasn't a better answer, I didn't yet know that is what was happening.

[every email you wrote me at the beginning ended saying:

remain in light, stop making sense];

Then you said write it in 10 words, not 9, or 11, or 13, 10 : exactly ; then,

50,   100,

200

Then we decided to work on *the bones*, the philosophical/imagery skeleton that would hold up the stories to be told. We needed to make sure I was being concise. The 51,000 words I wrote were not that and I never read it again after we started writing from emptiness.

You had me read Samuel R. Delany's "About 5,750 Words" :   I read :: *The red sun is high, the blue low.* A paragraph for every word aching with intentionality. Not one too many, nor one too little.

You said:

Write a chapter in 250 words. exactly.

I had just moved to Vancouver Island that week and was watching the sun set every night, taking in the unfolding cycles that have been in movement for 4.5 billion years. Time out of mind. I was falling in love with the cycle of the day, of day then night, life then death and resurrection. The cycle of my bipolar and soul. It was meant to be a vacation before settling into our new home but I was so moved by the sky and the Pacific Ocean. And by you, Sha.

I decided to write the *bones* in triptychs. Three 250-word sections, every morning for three weeks. We talked almost daily. You: asking me questions, expanding and contracting my writing and consciousness. On August 2, 2020, you sent me a rewrite of one of my sections described as a "Sha-ZAM" rewrite. I was laying on the beach watching my kids in the water, hot hot sun pressing on my skin, and what you sent me was an apocalypse

— a revelation that can only be known in its unfolding —

pure illumination, an event horizon that I passed through. There was so much pleasure in your writing, I could see how much you enjoyed being playful. Capitalizing entire words, using odd punctuation, breaking sentences into vertical lists. Like Michelangelo's unfinished sculptures I could see the form of the book bursting out of the rumble stone forged outside time. I started scratching at my arm as I read this 250-word passage and sketched it onto my bones, finding its way into my marrow. Then

absolute flow

I felt like I had a new language and began to feel out its boundaries spacing

: punctuation *italic passages*

lists for
poems
that would f
a
l
l

the keyboard << || >>
everything was possible. Writing was visual. Thank you, Sha

After three weeks the bones were done, and I started the stories, Iqaluit,
then cancer
then madness {{{{{{me and CAMH}}}}}
Every story you had me identify the beginning middle end.
You were this book's beginning. Brian came into its middle. I don't know when it will end. I'm having the press add an amendment to my contract so I can keep working on it after it is published.
—maybe a 1 of 1 artist book for you—

You are a radiant jewel, dear Sha.

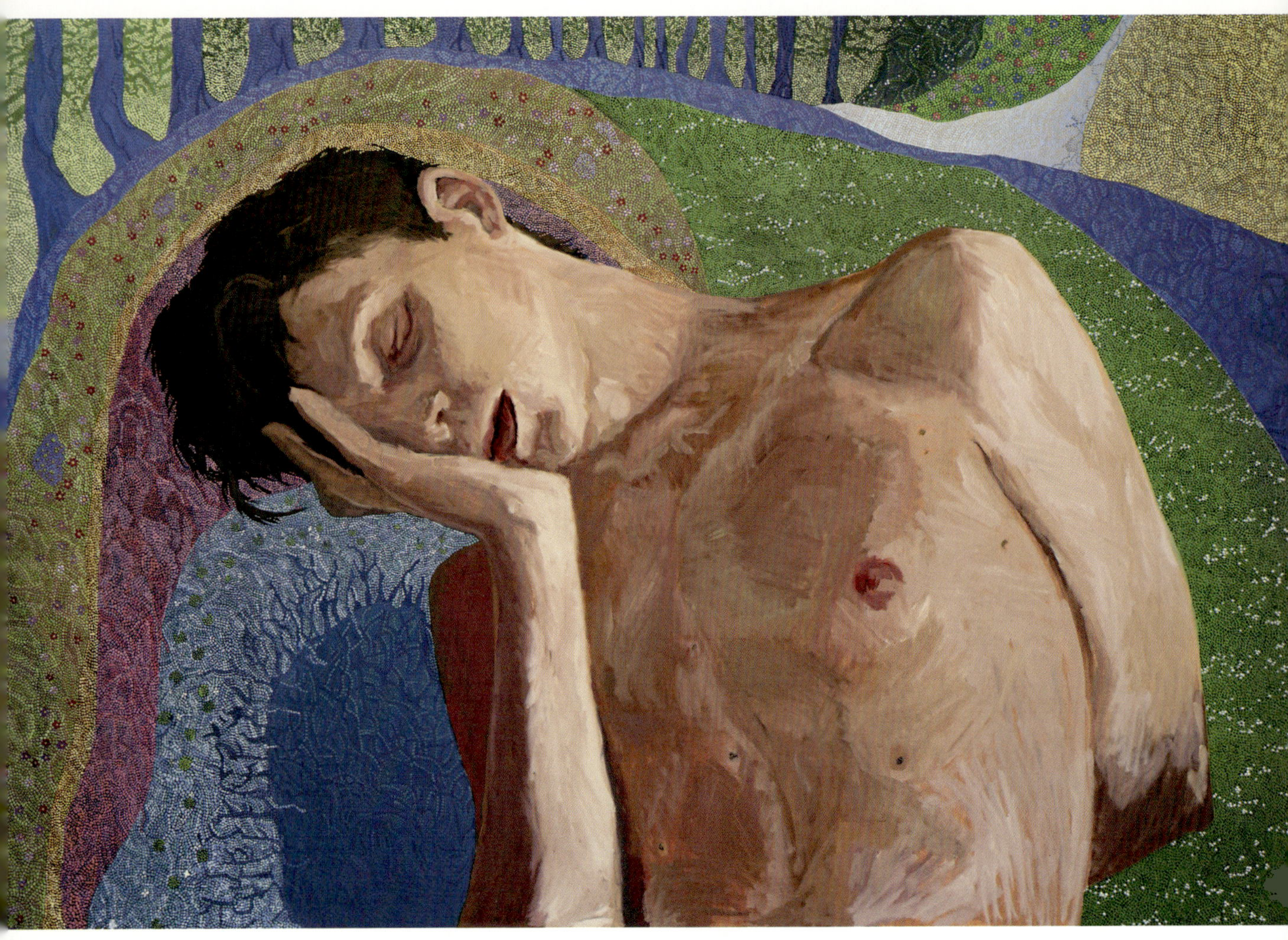

The Net of Jewels, 2021.
Oil painting on canvas,
3.3' × 5'.

INTRODUCTION

This is a story of a healing journey. Both mine and the people and communities I spent time with. I experienced trauma as a child and now I live with bipolar affective disorder: depression, mania, anxiety. All the people I met through my research were healing from trauma, whether in their childhood, cancer, or mental illness. And then I look at people across my life, and we are all trying to heal—to imagine new futures, hope new hopes, and feel whole, secure, and sustained.

Art is healing. //Art takes the ordinary and makes it extra-ordinary, it takes the everyday and makes it sacred //, it heightens experience and helps us *experience otherwise, story otherwise,* and make connections for complex meanings and understandings. Art is a fundamental human behaviour and every human can create, in their own way, and participate in art.

Much of these stories are about suffering. Many believe that suffering is the cause to bring about its end. It is where healing begins from. So there will be tough stories but there will also be stories of hope and healing. This story begins with suffering but it will end looking over the Pacific Ocean in a mental space I could have never imagined at the beginning of this journey. The process of conducting this research, creating the art, and writing this book has been the most healing period in my life. This is a healing manifesto.

For those who are suffering, I want you to see you are not alone. I also want you to know there is a *way through* the hurt. But it is not somewhere you end up, but a constant process of becoming and healing. And it is an amazing process to witness, to experience, to Be.

For those who are watching a loved one suffer, I want you to know their hurt is also your hurt. I have seen so many amazing people care, cry, *beat their hands at phantom walls*, and awaken to the experience of their loved ones. I have seen you want to trade places, take on the pain, even if just for a moment: relief. You are on a healing journey just as much as your loved one—you are in it together.

fieldwork

I spent five years being with people suffering.

We talked to each other, listened to each other, and hoped with each other. Then we co-created art together, uncovering stories of that suffering and where we wanted to go. These experiences changed my life.

I was in the beautiful community of Iqaluit, Nunavut, perched at the top of the world, *a land beyond the land*. A community struck by suicide, loss over loss, but full of Knowing and Spirit: hope. We made living sculptures of our bodies, imagining a way through this hurt.

I witnessed people recovering from head and neck cancer, a recovery that never ends. We created new stories of hope and healing together. I took videos of their injured faces, cut them up, made them swirl and roar, disintegrate, then recombine. I wanted them to know I saw their pain. They do not need to hide, they are seen.

I spent time with children in a psychiatric hospital in Toronto recovering from mental illness and addiction. Children with unbelievable pasts, now standing in a hospital painting a mural together, all the kids in a line, spilling paint and laughing, forgetting, for a moment, all the things that led them here—they were kids being kids. I saw myself as a child in that hospital.

Then I met Derek and Luanna in the throes of mania, up on the fifth floor of the Centre for Addiction and Mental Health. I learnt so much about mania, about recovery from you, and, four weeks after meeting you, I would reflect all of you through my mania. I still wonder what that recovery would have been like if we could have been together.

Then I look at the life I live and breathe, that brought me to all these places, to be with all these people, to experience their pain, to take on that pain, and try to make meaning out of that pain through art. The art we co-created, the art I made about those experiences, and now, the creation of this book, that itself summoned all of this pain but was the beginning of a marvellous gradient to flow upon; that was the most healing experience of my life. As these stories unfolded I found new ways to heal. It took five years of witnessing mental illness and recovery to teach me how to heal. But this isn't some endpoint, but a process, an awakening that continues

moment to moment, breath to breath, being to being *we are.*

research-creation

I employ research-creation methods to conduct artistic fieldwork with people and communities living with illness—witnessing, listening, caring, *falling, and merging*—co-creating art to make meaning from the experience of mental illness and recovery. The way my artistic and scholarly practice engages with research-creation is through the provocation of *creation-as-research*: the act of creation is a site of knowledge generation and meaning-making. Co-creating with people is creation-as-research. Bringing these works and stories into my own practice and freely expressing the sensations and insights that arise from engaging those works is creation-as-research.

From these open and intuitive gestures, I created paintings, photographs, videos, films, a play, and creative texts for exhibitions, film festivals, theatre productions, publications, and public readings. Presenting this work publicly creates a safe, inclusive space for those with illness to feel validated, to feel seen, and, hopefully, to feel less alone. And for those who have not met these experiences to empathetically engage with the possibility of that experience.

The conversations, tears, and smiles I have experienced sharing this work over the years have changed my life. I didn't yet understand how much.

I began this text with Sha LaBare and we believe research-creation creates space for scholarly research to be told in *other* ways—a lived, affective, creative expression of fieldwork, philosophy, and the life that lived and breathed that research, how I shaped the research and it shaped me. How research-creation can weave and knot author, subject, environment, and spirit into a singular net: Being.

structure

This is a nonlinear unfolding but I hope to have placed many wayfinding elements: dates, places, mental states, alternative table of contents, and the Notes on Conditions. If you find an unknown term or turn of phrase, it will very likely be described in the Notes on Conditions at the end of the book with a further section of direct references back to the source material. I recommend you quickly flip back to it to see what it holds. For instance, early sections, such as *Telling Stories Otherwise*, have many key words used throughout the book that the Notes on Conditions could aid in opening awarenesses to the intent of these words.[1]

With these aids, I hope you can find your way through this journey.

Note

1. Now look at the Notes on Conditions for this Introduction on page 235, it's written for ~~you~~.

Today, I want to think through those who came before me and after me
—about family, heredity, and
what I call
the open.
I also want to think about genetically passed down altered states and their relation to
Being and Time.

To begin, I'm going to tell a story, or a series of stories, about some experiences with time I am having.

✳ November 2017: I am sitting beside a pool on a rooftop in Arizona. I'm looking at the scar that stretches from one side of my pelvis to the next as I write. I don't remember the day I got it, but I sense it. I sense it with a deep hunger, turning three, days before. After the surgery, I am not allowed to eat for ten days as my large intestine grows back together. The nurses would give me popsicles only to have them pumped back out through a nose feeding tube that runs into my stomach:
sensations in my nose,
at the back of my throat,
choking on
tubes.

This scar makes me think of my mother. While it might be on my body, it's her scar too. The years we spent in
waiting rooms,
doctor's offices,
(pain on the bedroom floor)
and hospital rooms.

Time doesn't move in those rooms. You look out the window and people are going in and out of buildings, trying to be on time. In here there is no time. You have the beeping of the machines, but measures like day and night, breakfast and supper, 4 and 5 p.m. don't exist. Melancholy time exists as my mother is grieving her child, a child that is only a few feet away from her, but one whose potentiality, whose futures are depleting.

✳ Psychiatric hospital. Toronto.
May 2017: I meet Derek and I think he works at the hospital.
He is very pleasant, well-spoken, and approachable.

I feel like I know him, or have known him, like I'd know him if I remembered hard enough. His glasses look broken and his ability to hold eye contact was flickering. In this moment, I care deeply for him, like a brother. But there is a sense that maybe he is me.

It's something I don't understand yet.

I don't hesitate in becoming close with Derek.

We share a madness experience,

coarse and twisting,   knotting,

stringing along a stretching expanse.

It's not just the physical trace expressed in our genomes,

suggesting some still present common ancestor, but transitory:

we are all there, somewhere unconcealed, but not always accessible.

✳ For me, illness is not a catastrophe, and it isn't simply about making-better or curing, but is a species-level meaning-making event. Illness is a very ancient space and we all inhabit it. It's nested deep within each of us, deeper than the genetic strands stretching across a geological timescale of billions of years; it is a space for communal immunitary kinship, where our bodies heal the gnawing of

microscopic predators,

genetic expressions,

{madness},,,

and time.

When I have my children, I become intensely aware—deeper than in an embodied way, more like a geological awareness, long and vast and much closer to the ground than I ever thought I could be—of all the illnesses that marked my life.

In the winter of 2016, I am standing in front of my great-grandparents' graves reading to them about their daughter, in a land I haven't been to before, and a flash of lightning places me both before and after, an intergenerational being, and I wonder

:: who am I from and who am I to? ::

I become present to my place in a vast line of parents who have all died,

and to that, somehow,

I must learn how to die as a parent.

✳ *"Don't forget Paraskevia (Smokey Lake) where your ancestors are buried,"* reads a note attached to a picture taken in the 1990s, in Smokey Lake, Alberta. The picture shows my father and my paternal grandparents, with their backs to the graves of my great-grandparents. I visit this site and the gravestone remains new—shiny black marble, etched with names and dates.

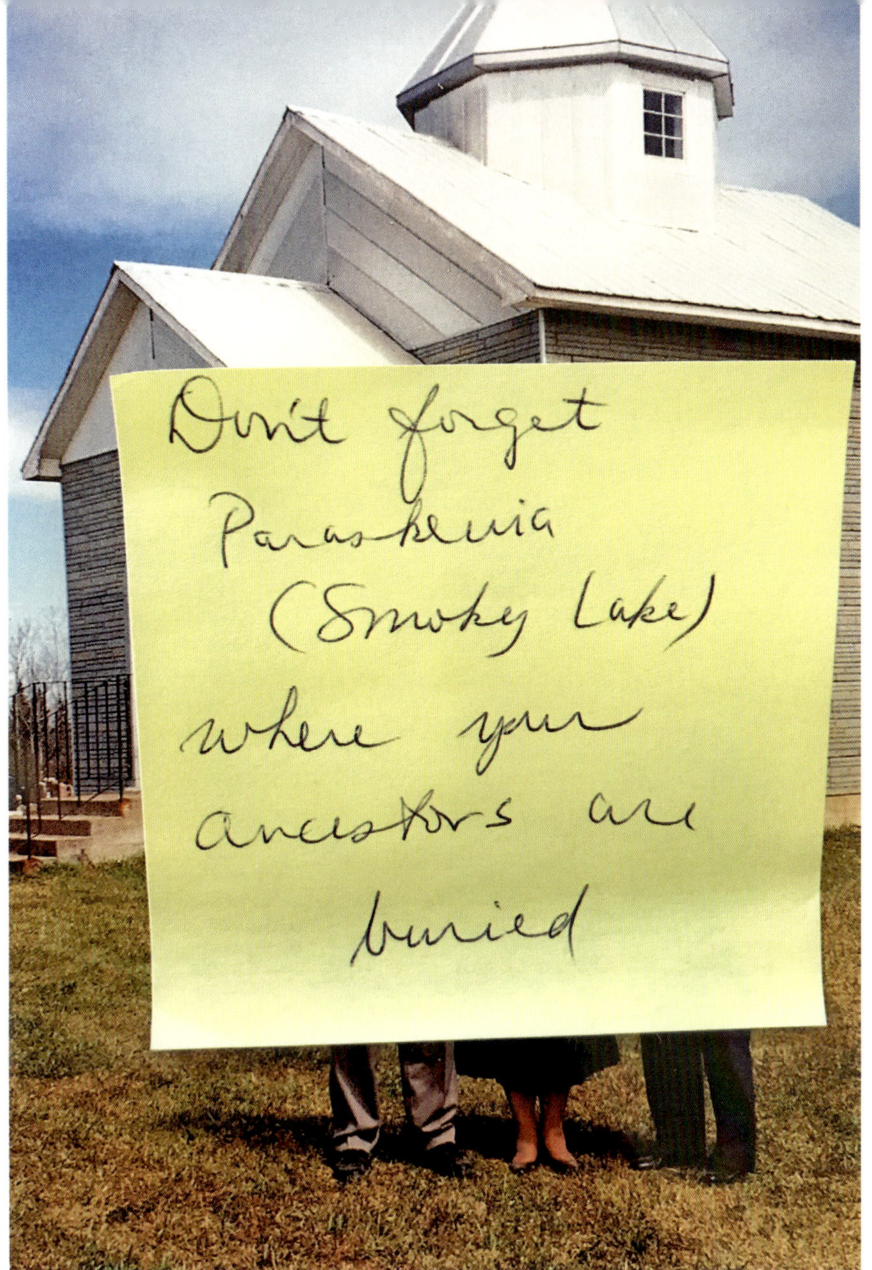

A note. Sometime ago.

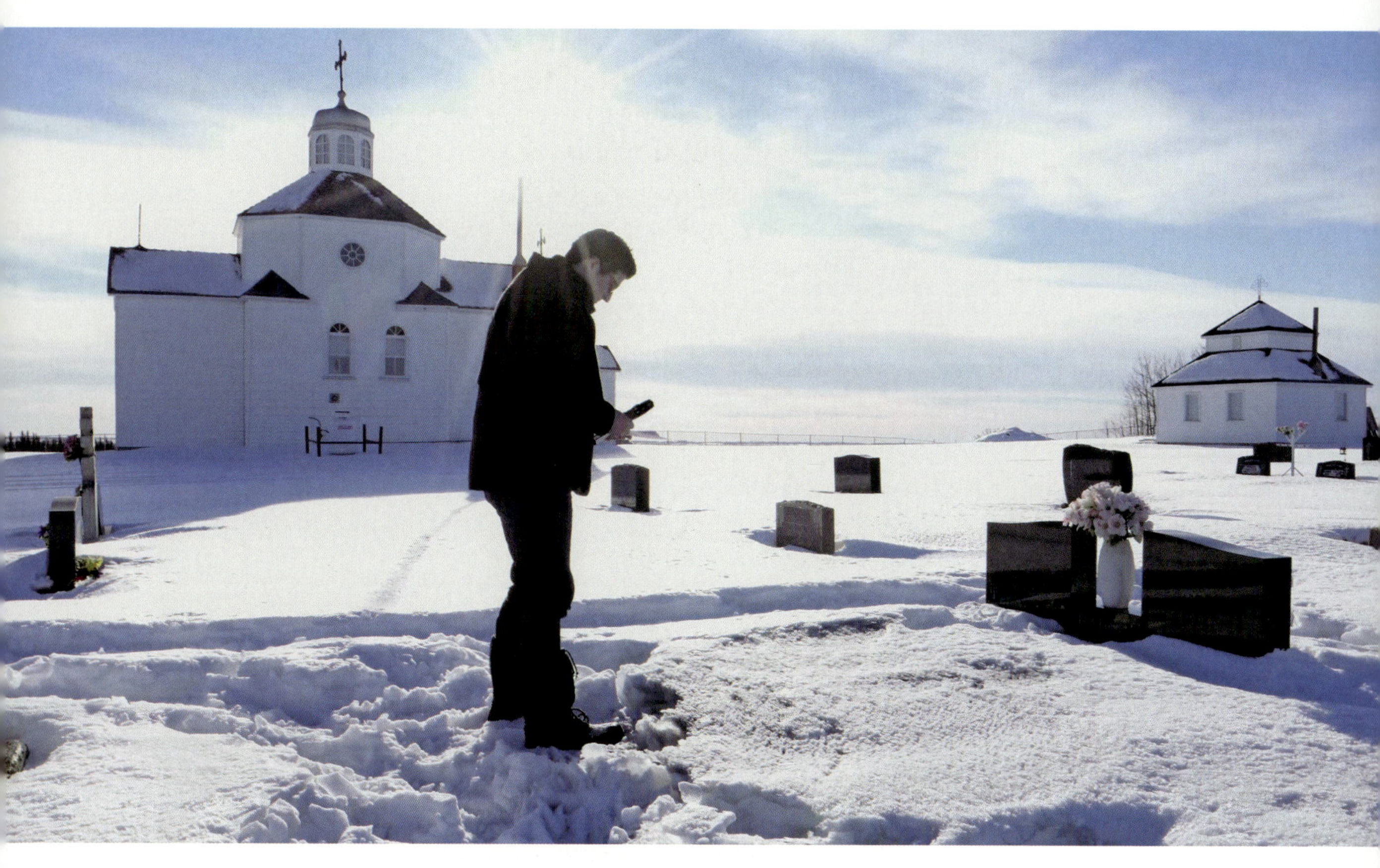

Paraskevia Church and graveyard, Smokey Lake, Alberta, January 2016.

The new stones were put in on the day of that photo, to replace the worn stone from their Ukrainian funeral, etched by wind and time. When I get this photograph, the note obscures all three figures, leaving only the surrounding space of the graveyard, a place at once familiar

(I had seen this image, or one like it, before)

and yet strange, made so by the effacement of paper and words: *this is where your ancestors are buried*.

✳ Watching my daughter's hair lighten to a fair blonde, considering her crisp blue eyes, and seeing the ultrasound photographs of her malformed kidney, I can't help but remember something: a woman I have never met until finding her nested in my daughter, my maternal grandmother. I never had any pull to her until I watch her son die, Ellie become ill, and the near miscarriage of my second daughter.

(Did she ever miscarry?)

I want to understand her at one point, and then, at another point, I don't want to understand her anymore. Instead, I am trying to understand myself, to make room in myself for my role as a father.

✳ I first receive this photograph with the note on it, I don't think much of it. My aunt has always been intergenerational, sending me odd notes and pictures, so I just put it to the side. However, for years, including a move to a new house, I never remove it from my desk. It stays piled amongst the ever-changing table refuse ,,, it's always there.

In the winter of 2016, it brings me to my paternal great-grandparents' graves, accompanied by my father. On the first trip, we find our way to the "Necyk" farm, one that was sold over seventy years ago, and speak to the current farmer. Talking with him about the farm's history, we can tell that the farmer cares deeply for this land.

He takes us on a drive through the fields.

My father tells us that his grandmother had a miscarriage in these fields.

In that moment, I experience time, ahead, then long and behind.

nine months later,

a bleed, the near miscarriage of Mary

A hundred years before

my great-grandma, terror in those fields,

loss, grief. Grieving a child, never kissed.

I didn't understand that yet.

My father asks if there is still a pile of rocks in the centre of the farm. The farmer takes us there. My father explains that the farm assigned to my great-grandfather when he brought his family from Ukraine was a field full of rocks—glacial rocks collecting, then dropping across a geological epoch. It would take him years to clear the field, each year slowly revealing more land to farm—generational time. Seeing that sculpture of rocks struck me. I feel my great-grandfather's labour, frustrations, and | time |. I can see how my grandfather never went into farming and became a school teacher.

Later, my father and I visit his mother's parents' graves.

There is an area off from the gravesite, deep within trees, for unnamed, unbaptized babies and people who died by suicide. The graves are so worn you couldn't read any of the names, and no one had replaced them, unlike my great-grandparents' graves. I wonder if they were my relatives.

(With this disorder the statistical odds of me dying by suicide are incredibly high.)

I walk up to the top of a small hill and, on that crisp winter day, I can see for miles. I see the rail line that my ancestors would have come on from Ukraine.

I see a great many things that aren't yet visible.

✳ In September of 2016, I begin to think about my unknown grandmother, who I assume is still alive. My maternal grandfather has been dead for years now and I still haven't cried for him.

I wonder what my grandmother would think of his death. She knows about it because she is close to one of my cousins who would have told her. I wonder what their love looked like, before they did all those tough things to each other.

I think more of Spedden, Alberta, the hamlet I started writing about years ago. I promise myself that I need to go there to film and for myself to see this land, and slowly I start to see the relationship between this place and the woman I will never meet. I won't.

I write about both of them, the place and the woman.

I write about the deep sadness I feel trying to hold all these things in my life together, and I could see how she was not able to.

I think of my bipolar diagnosis years ago.

(Would she have had the same diagnosis?)

People say that when they see Elliot, they see my mother.

Last weekend, at my brother's wedding, my cousin, the one who is in contact with my grandmother, says my mother looks identical to her mother. There is a photograph of my seven-month-old mother sitting in a bath in the kitchen sink smiling. Her mother left a few months before.

How did my grandfather take care of those four children alone? His family lived in Saskatoon.

Who would have helped him? I have no idea where his parents are buried.

I imagine myself alone with my children. Mary is now the age of my mother in that photograph.

Would she smile at me without her mother?

(Would I still be here?)

This last month, Candace and I take Elliot off her daily antibiotics, meant to prevent infections from overtaking her kidneys.

You had kidney problems.

My mother had kidney problems.

So did two of my cousins on my mother's side.

What else of you, Grandma, is nested in my daughters?

✳ In the summer of 2017, I'm in rural Pennsylvania writing about a different you, thinking about you, being with you: Derek.

Are you doing well?

Are you still out there?

I'm talking to a five-year-old child named Holden as he swims in the outdoor pool where I have my feet cooling. He wants to know what I am writing.

I say

I am trying to remember something.

He asks

when did it happen?

I say

a few months ago.

He asks

don't you just remember?

I say I am trying to.

✳ June 2017: I go manic three weeks after I leave you, Derek. It's the worst episode of my life.

I think of you often during that month. I wonder what my recovery would have looked like if we could have been together.

It was so lonely.

Remember when we went to the music room on that last day?

I record your hands as you improvise on the piano. Your voice is captivating.

That day you are returning down, slowing, and coming to realize all the things you have been through.

It looks painful,

you are losing control,

but it is part of your journey.

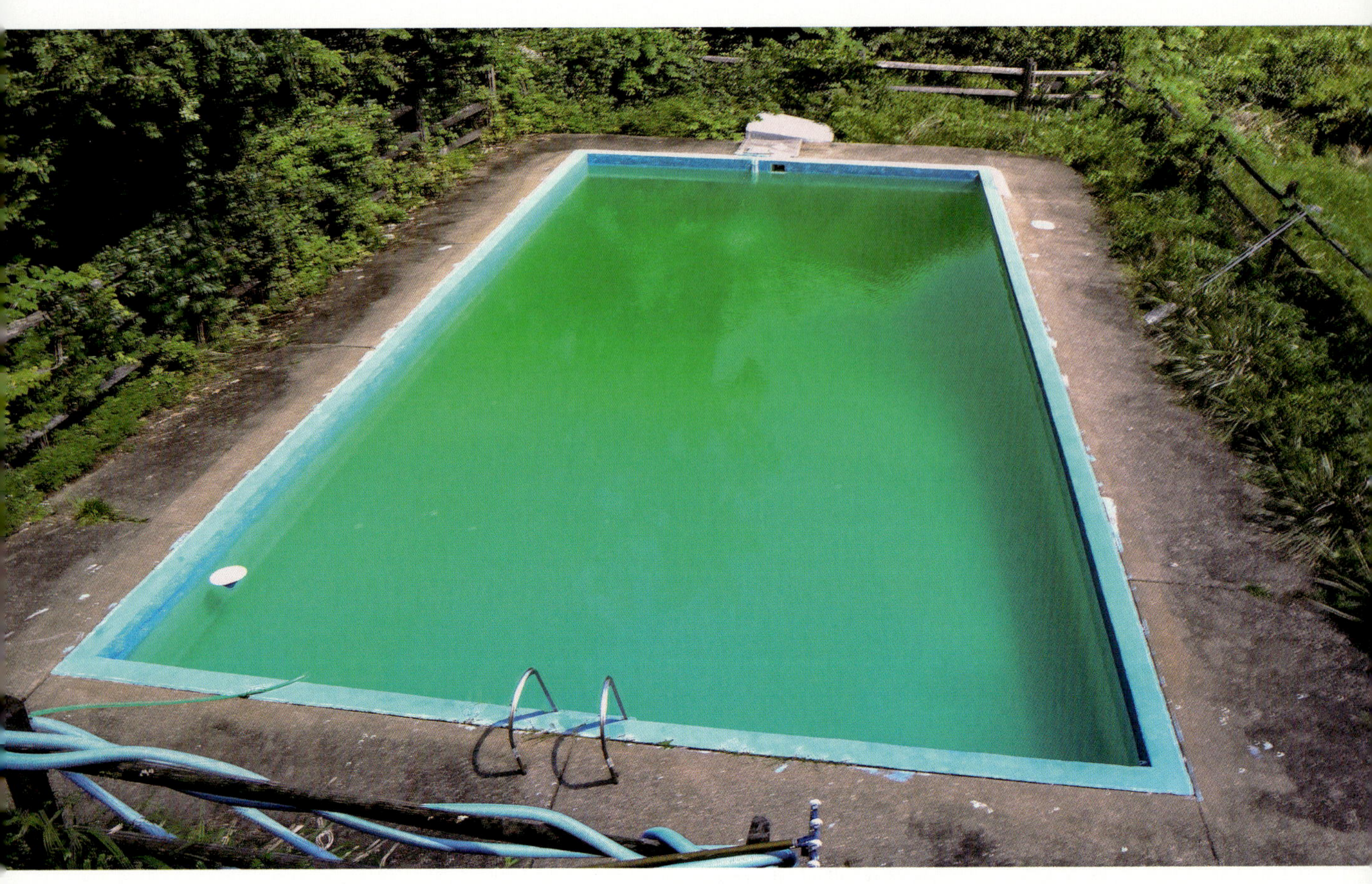

Rural Pennsylvania.
August day, 2017.

It isn't until I myself break that I am able to start putting all these experiences back together.

✳ I think of you, my daughters. How many things I want to share with you, and how I won't be what I am now but will be much older when that day comes.

I'm sitting on a small sofa bed in Greenwich Village,
New York City,
August 11, 2017,
11:46 p.m.,
33 years old,
watching a documentary about Bob Dylan with my dad.
This is the first time we share this experience together: sharing Dylan.
He is 66. Two years before Parkinson's, then stroke.

✳ June 18, 2017: I don't have any distinct memories from the previous two days. I know I took my pills, read a lot, and painted.

Today, I wake up and go downstairs.
Mary is crying, and I can tell that Candace
is exhausted
from being up with the girls
multiple times last night.
I mutter with hate to her
why did we have kids?
Candace shuts down and starts to cry.

Then, Elliot asks me for one of those small boxes of cereal that you can pour milk into and eat directly from.

I try to open it with my fingers,
then a knife,
but I can't open it because I'm
crying too hard.
Candace rushes me up to the bedroom. I keep crying.
Elliot
three-year-old Ellie, child
comes in and asks me what is wrong.
Candace says I hurt my leg but that I will be okay.
Elliot places a stuffy in my hand and Candace leaves me to cry.
slipping time, Candace comes back in:
we talk about many things, things that I don't want to remember saying.
Things no one should ever say.

I don't know how long I stay there. I hear Candace call my mom, herself crying, and asks for help. Soon, I hear them come in the front door. Candace comes up and asks me if I want to kill myself, and I say

I can't be left alone.

I fall asleep for many hours.

I awake with Candace by me. She asks if I am okay. I feel drained yet somehow better.

I tell her I hate myself for what I said.

It is Father's Day and I can't remember the faces of my children.
My parents are watching them downstairs as Candace and I are on the
bed upstairs.
I can't see anything anymore. All clarity is gone, and I am without affect.

I don't remember the rest of the day, but I know I take my pills that night.

✳ Sometime in the dream, my dad drives me to the university to see my friend, Dan Harvey. I lay out several papers I want to write with him.

Cancer Madness Anthropocene
pain pain pain

He listens.
I know I'm not making complete sense, but he listens anyway.
As we sit outside a hard rain hits and we rush inside.
We talk, but I am looking out the window.
Did it always rain this hard?
I become intensely aware of my body being pulled
down
and
down
onto our planet.
I feel the rotation of the earth, the momentum around the sun,
the weight of Jupiter, then
around the centre of the galaxy,
and of the pull of everything toward everything
within the supercluster of galaxies we are within.
I feel the abyss
a million lifetimes
colder than cold. (I gaze in)
Dan and I still talk.
I realize there is no place to escape, that I am stuck in this husk of flesh
on a rocketing planet,
in an indifferent universe.
Why am I not getting the ecstatic revelations, the communions with god that Derek got?

Why is mine so meaningless and devoid of hope?
(I don't understand yet)

I find my dad sleeping in the car in a parking lot. We come home, and I continue to paint.

✳ I finally eat.

My mind is too fast, and I think I'm going to throw up.

I am dizzy, not the kind that would make you fall but the kind that unbalances your soul.

I tell Candace about this, and she sends me to the pharmacy to fill my antipsychotic medication. She suspects I am in a manic episode and I will have to slow myself down with drugs.

In the pharmacy, there are aisles and aisles of
ordered and repeated objects
of care: deodorant toothpaste tampons
As I walk through the aisles and aisles
my visual experience falls out of sync

with the standard seamlessness of my visual field,
and time itself, becomes a falsity,
a grand illusion.

reality—

Walking down that aisle time becomes a
flat disc,
where everything that was or would be rotates for infinity, and I
would be in that aisle forever
<I have dreamt of this aisle, had dreamt, dream of this aisle>
Driving home the sky opens,
and the crisp blue prairie sky takes on a new vibrancy,
and just then every generation of my ancestors sees it too,
and I, an intergenerational being
—make kinship with everyone before,
and with all my children's children's children.
We all share this sky.

✳ I take my medications and sleep that night.

I wake up and can't focus my eyes.

I go downstairs and my family,
my children,
are not mine anymore, not my own.
I think back to Sunday, to wondering about how many pills I'd have to take to die.
That's when Candace calls my parents for help.
They come, and I feel ashamed.
My dad goes into the garage to look at my paintings. He turns to me and cries and holds me.

It is me crying   holding an adult Elliot.
I see a thousand of my ancestors crying,
but then I realize the physicality of my father's body.
He's getting old.
His control over the world, over his children, over his body|mind, is waning.
I feel so sad that he sees me this way.
Then I fall into the VISION
Ellie   O, Mary.
worlds one,   growing closer
knotting   weaving
strung   cosmic expanse
common ancestor   god // I love you.
and I am so scared that I will have to hold you like my father is holding me now.
I tell him I will   get better.
I finish the large painting.
I see Derek.
I see his broken glasses, how similar he and I look,
I feel the wear on his notebook and see his gentleness, his intellect.
He is twelve years older than me and has been hospitalized six times before.
I thought my life would be different, but a month after meeting him I'm here, now, in this room, with these pills, drinking them down, thinking about how to get it done.
How to kill myself.
I think of my ancestors, stretching back into the Holocene and before.
What did their love look like?
Did they have children with my diseases|disorders?
Did they grieve them?
What was it like for them to hold their children, their child?
I think forward to my children, and their children, and their children's children.

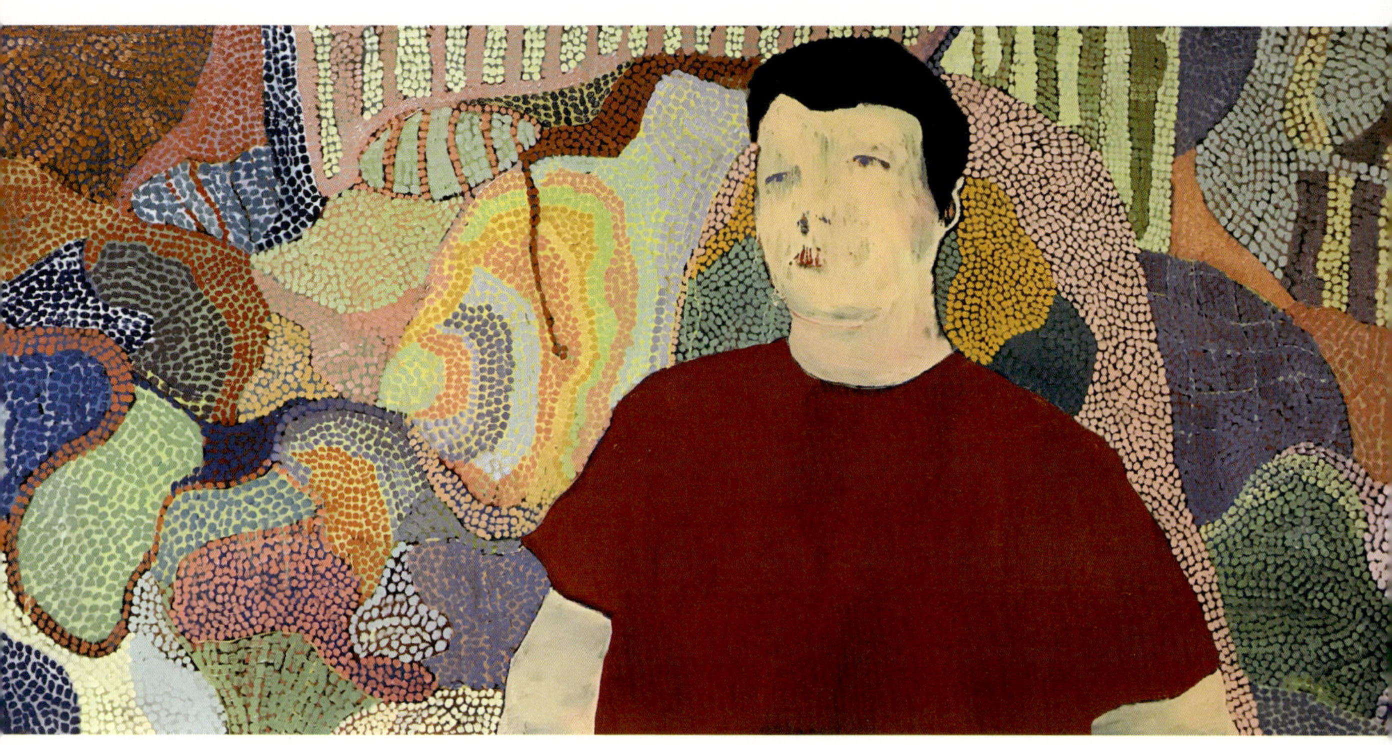

Mania, 2017. Oil painting on canvas, 3.5' × 7'.

I feel the world in pain,
a geological pain.
I feel eco-sickness as I breathe in the smoke from the forest fires
in the north
west
east
south.
I feel eco-anxieties as a rain hits one that hits particularly hard,
that pours over my gutters
and breaks my ancient elm tree.
What will their world be like?
How could I have brought them into this?
I feel intense guilt.
In 2046 Elliot will be my age now. Mary 2049.
They will have first-hand experience of a natural disaster,
the loss of everything in everything everywhere.
What impact will that have on their psyche?
Will these eco-traumas begin an epigenetic cascade into a bipolar episode?
Will I hold Ellie, Mary like my father holds me?

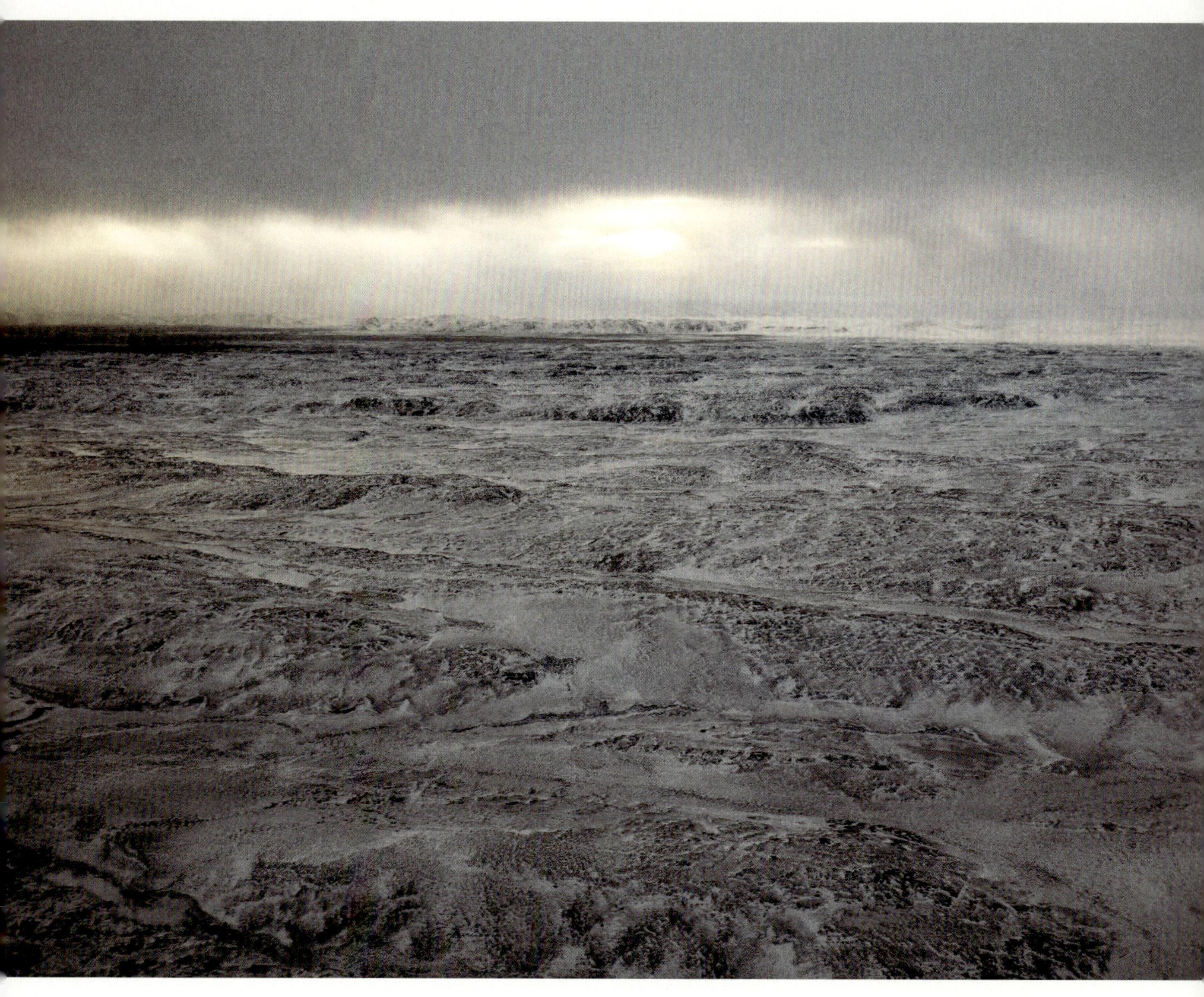

Landing in Iqaluit, Nunavut, late October 2016.

breathe in
breathe out

I'm not much of a traveller.

Red-eye from Edmonton, 30 minutes in Toronto, flickering sleep in the Ottawa airport, retrofitted for cargo Boeing 747 heading for Iqaluit: the only capital city in Canada not accessible by road.

Strange flight. Only four rows at the front for people, then a wall with cargo behind. People with bottles of vodka in their bags talking about the conference. I keep to myself. The flight wasn't bumpy but the plane seemed to follow a sine wave:

up and up
then slipping
down and down.

I have my laptop on my legs: building slides. I have no idea what I'm doing. *Where* I'm going. I type the title:

"Writing Suicide"

What do I know about that, other than my own? I wrote about it two times for Elliot in artworks. The slides are empty. Computer on lap, warming and losing power.

We slip, then slip
Pilot: *flight attendants, prepare for landing*.
Knowing he means: and so we fall, *because falling is easier than resisting*.

I gaze out the windows on both sides of the plane,
looking at clouds from both sides now.
Humming Joni Mitchell in my mind.
What do I know about clouds at all?

Fall: out of the misting dreams of heaven, revealing a sensation across a vast stark landscape. Round, stunted mountains of black breaking through untouched snow. There is something missing, the roots of the world, the giving essence of this planet, there is an absence:

no soil, grass, bushes, or trees
anywhere.

A barren Martian landscape, without the red. Lunar black and grey compressed by white misting clouds.

I am t

here.

As I step off the plane, I'm enveloped in Arctic air. Frobisher Bay, just over that black and white hill. Flickering awareness:

Ovid's signpost laying bare:

BEYOND HERE LIES NOTHING. A land beyond the land. Chillness, hostility, frozen waves of an ice-hard sea.

Ovid has lost his hope, but something here has not.

I walk across the tarmac towards the airport. Brightly coloured, prefabricated modular units, brought here from somewhere else, another land beyond the land.

NO CELL SERVICE.

I should have written down the hotel's address. No one to call. Where am I again?

Okay

breathe in breathe out

I'm not much of a traveller.

I step off the tarmac, up a ramp and into the single room airport. I'm tired, and this building is tired, too. I step out the other side, snow, a taxi loop. Then into a van:

can you take me into town?

seven dollars.

We leave the loop, turn onto a road, around the hill, pull to the side of the road. Three minutes.

welcome to Iqaluit.

I get out and look at my cell. Rogers Extended Network. Two bars. Email: hotel just across the snowed-in street.

October 26, 2016.

4:27 p.m: sunset. City lights.

I look to my right ;;; hotel.

In front, tire tracks to some scattered buildings and Frobisher Bay: chain-linked fences, buildings collapsing into the snow, frozen ships, and *the ice-hard sea*...

I look to my left, four-storey buildings on stilts: weathering the Arctic climate, avoiding heat transfer. Further up a hill, lights flicker on. Prefabricated homes shaped like submarines or research outposts. None of this stuff is from here, it all comes from somewhere else.

I turn around to nothing but snow and darkness. No signpost necessary.

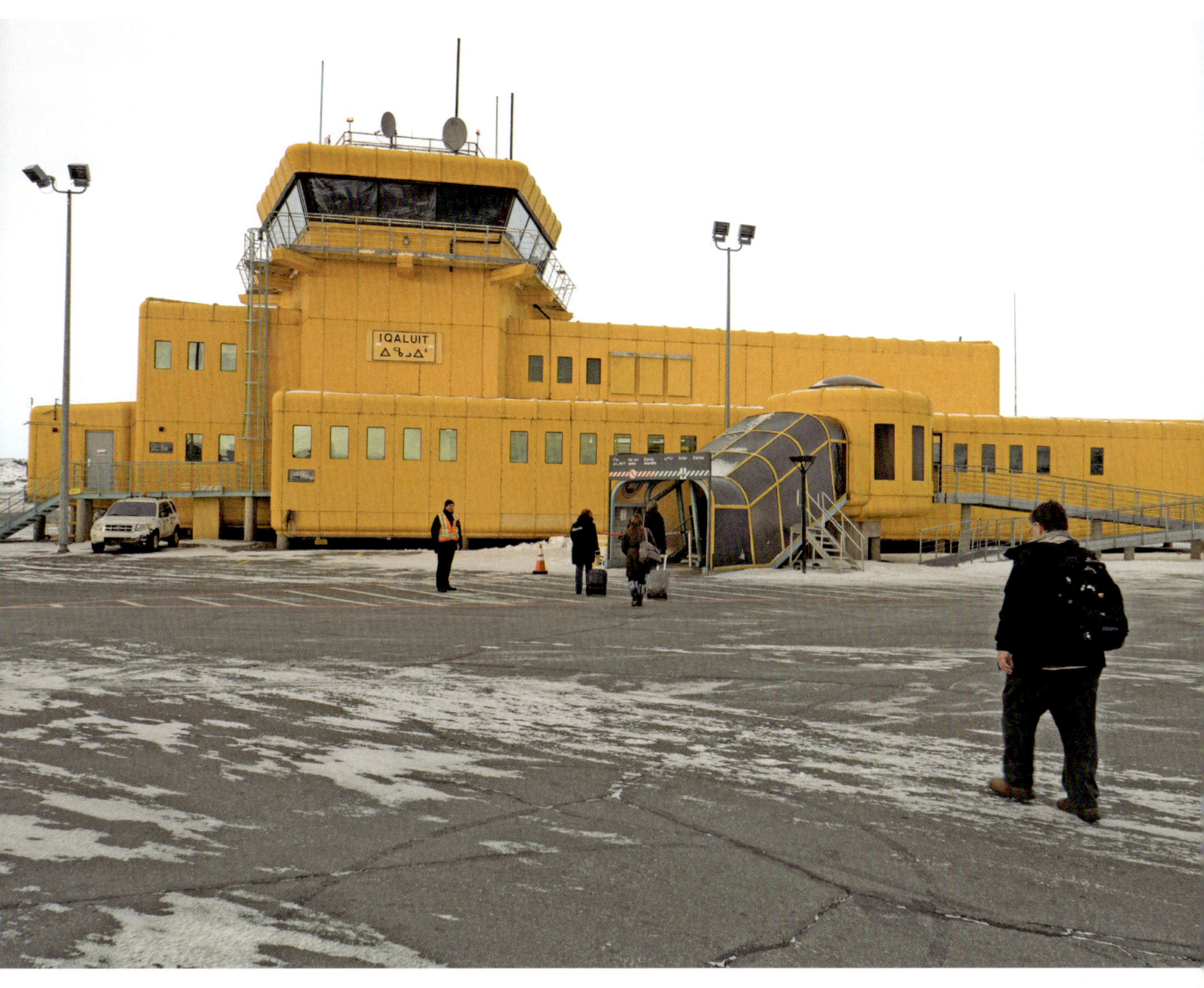

Former Iqaluit Airport,
late October 2016.

NOTHING

I walk into the hotel and fall into my room. I lay on the bed thinking about the red-eye flight. Thinking about teaching at MacEwan University 24 hours ago, then driving to the University of Alberta and teaching a night class. Then, 10 p.m.: eating pizza in the sculpture studio with my two TAs. Feeling anxious about the trip ahead of me: travel, travail.

I gaze back further, in my mind. I think of my Indigenous grandma, Grandma Rogers. I remember she adopted my mom as a child. Raised by her and my grandpa with her three brothers and a stepsister with another brother to come seven years later.

My mom said my grandma would walk six feet behind her dad.

An Indian only follows.

Sadness.

My mind slips to going up north, near the Alberta/Northwest Territories border: Paddle Prairie. Where my grandma was raised. Where she left. Only for a while.

I feel my body shrink to the size I was as a kid, sitting around the fire, thirty people, staying up past my bedtime, listening to my family play guitar and sing country and folk songs. Wow, can my family play and sing!

My mind gazes back to my Grandpa Necyk, playing the fiddle, speaking Ukrainian.

All part of something larger and longer. Expressing and unfolding.

I feel my way back into my body, behind my eyes. Across the room is a blistering colourful painting: Inuit. Something conceals, pressing on my Being.

Damn you Canada.

The Canada then, but also now, still now.

Assimilation.

Acculturation.

Trauma. Death.

A deadly government that set in motion all the events that lead me here for a conference on suicide. Here because Iqaluit has the worst suicide rate in Canada,

one of the highest in the world.

Not yet unconcealed to me, it hangs in the room.

Suffering is the cause to bring about its end; through suffering, we come to Know ourselves.

I look at a painting created by someone in this city. Decoration in a hotel, sure, but written in a language of Knowing and Spirit. I sit up and squint at the details. I should probably just put on my glasses.

My mind is full of colour as I turn to stand in an art exhibition from a few years before: Professor Gavin Renwick, Canada Research Chair in Design Studies, University of Alberta. He taught me things I wasn't yet ready to understand: waiting for alignment. Showing a series of drawings of government-designed houses that would be built for the Indigenous Peoples of the North over decades, he whispers to me through them:

Notice how the landscape itself seems to actively resist external architecture and control, whether through cold, lack of materials, or desire. How can we say the people and the land are separate? Distinctions where there are no distinctions.

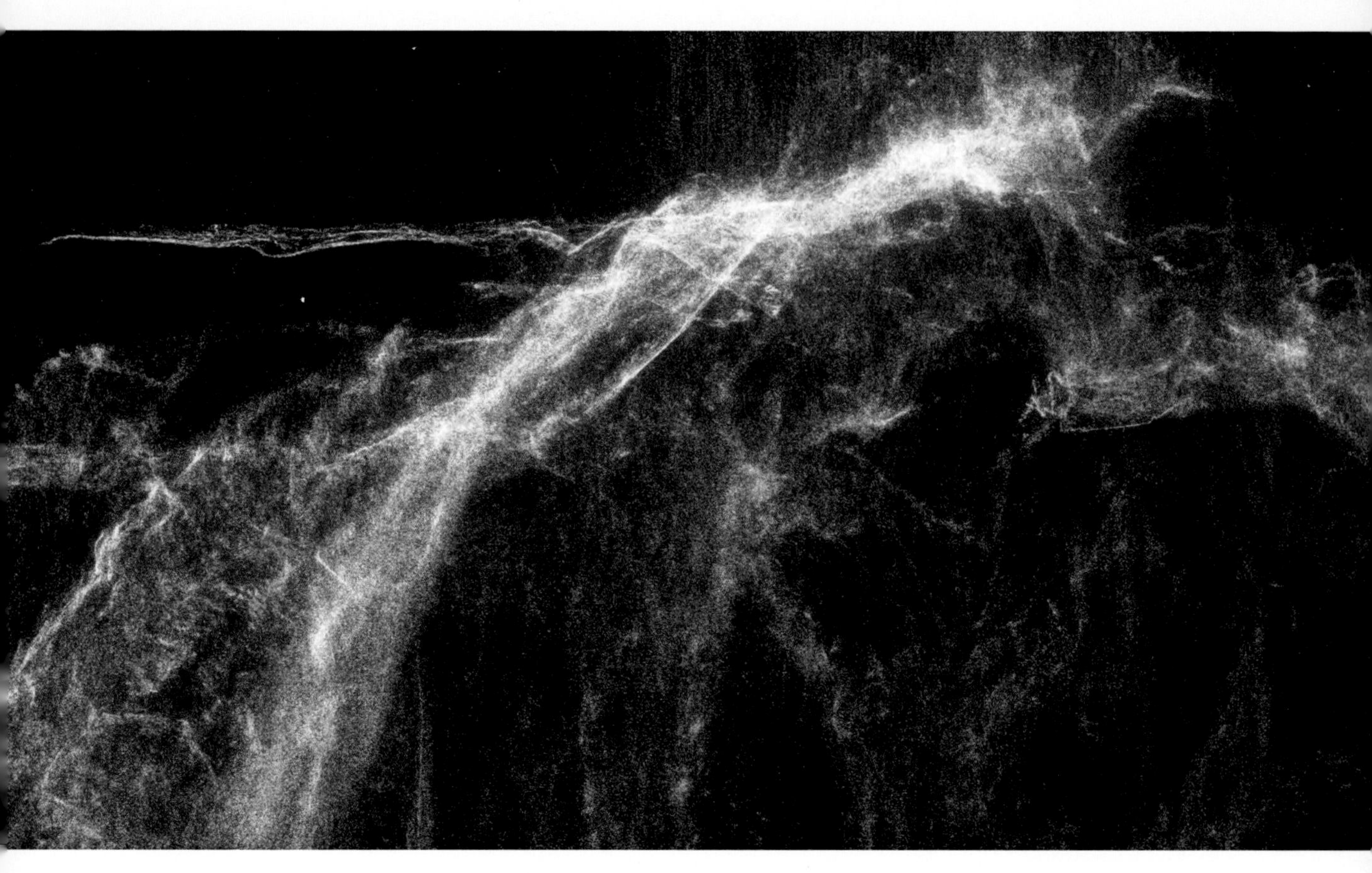

Kingdom of Illumination (breath), 2020. 18-minute video created with Gary James Joynes.

These are all stories. Stories of suffering, illness, healing, philosophy, spirituality, and visionary art. Stories

— *// all the way down. //*

Stories told by an artist, lived experiences that provoke my practice and my Being. They are as factual and as vulnerable as I know how to make them, and I mean them as provocations for your healing journey.

I am on my journey and you are on yours.

But we are in this together.

Thomas King, storyteller and radiant light, ends his stories by saying:

> *// It's yours. Do with it what you will. Tell it to friends. Turn on a television movie. Forget it. But don't say in the years to come that you would have lived your life differently if only you had heard this story.*
>
> *You have heard it now. //*

Storying otherwise is what we bring back from our exchange with *the abyss*, stories of our new orientation that bleed into the waking world, lucid dreaming. There is nothing to be reasoned, nothing to think through, this is not about intellect, just about Knowing—the unconcealment of Being. Stories otherwise are heightened accounts in the presence of Being—full of heaven and hell, with life and death hung in the room, blasting with primordial imagery and pure affective experience that radiate inwards not noticing your skin or the mental boundaries you've erected, and bursting forth with expression: gestures to the abyss.

The visionary artist is a storyteller otherwise, bringing back these field notes. Visionary art is a world that personal and collective suffering inhabits so that it can start, we can start healing, becoming.

We cling to our Self like it's life or death, and find a Charon to cross over, with:

visions | *madness* | *psychedelics* | *meditation*

We create space for spaciousness, inviting in the abyss—the mother of all muses. It's nonrational, nonlinguistic, nonlinear, with layered meanings, in flux, and on the verge of disintegration. These properties imprint on the vision-seeker and the fallen field recordings, visionary art, take on these same properties. Stories otherwise from this space, orientations to Being, lift the veil of the world and create glimpses into the open, before the abyss.

And, as Nietzsche says, when you gaze long into an abyss, it gazes into you.

A relationship is forged, a portal is open, and an exchange unfolds.

In this space, the vision-seeker makes a gesture. And with luck, the abyss makes a gesture back.

Sending a sensation up your spine,
into your mind,
cracking open consciousness,
making space for spaciousness within,
a clearing before Being.

Or it may present itself, stand before you and show you primordial images from your ancestral heritage. It might show you

the beginning of the universe
your birth or your death
the monsters that plague you in your dreams or throughout your childhood
yourself, plain as day, with no filter or comforting hallucination, provoking you to experience that you are nobody
fractal patterns of the quantum field of the world-out-there reflecting in Indra's Net in every direction in the infinite psychic space of the conscious universe
God
that you are God
It may bathe you in love or wound you in hatred.

All of these are provocations, deep sensations forcing you to express yourself, *to grow closer* to the abyss. And so you do, and you show some more of yourself. The abyss watches. It witnesses. You are seen. You world the abyss in place and the abyss worlds you. It's an exchange. It reveals you both, unconceals you both, allows you both to be simultaneously witnessed. To be seen. To Be.

We need to heal. Let us heal. The perils facing humanity and the more-than-human world cannot be met with technology, science, or rationality. To forge a way forward we need new and ancient stories, healing stories. We need a

;;;Knowing:::

from the abyss, so we can experience, sense, and promise new worlds and futures—new ways to *Be*.

This is the work of a visionary artist. We are the seers, mystics, healers, who go down and bring back orientations to Being, and we communicate them through stories otherwise—*the world of a visionary artwork*.

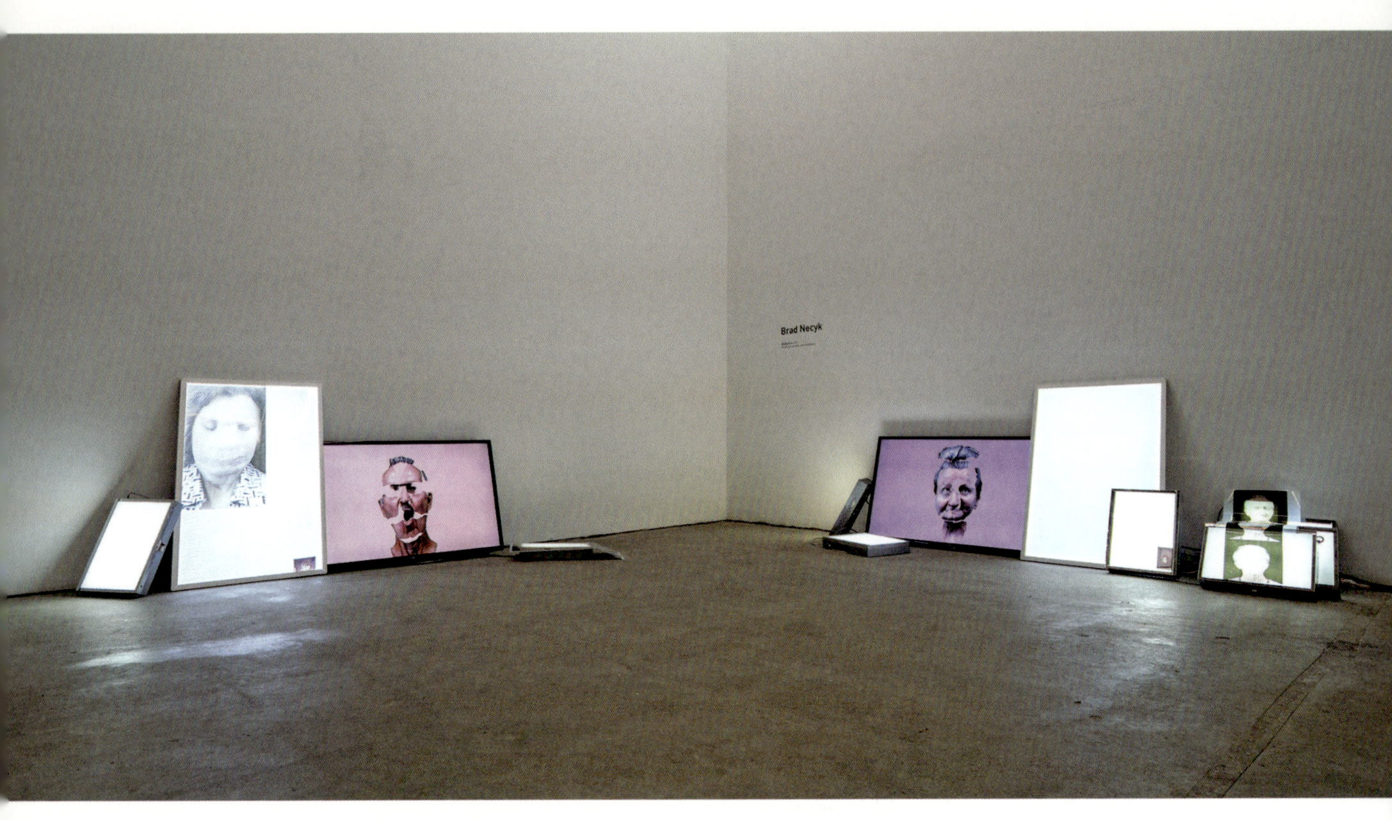

Installation, dc3 Art Projects in Edmonton, Alberta, January 2017.

UNIFIED PALE, PINK BACKDROPS the cluster of coloured facial markings,
cheek, lips, chin, eye, forehead.

Marks in the air that swirl, scream, overlap; untethered to one another... restless, yet almost colliding, to make something whole, something usable. But always on the surface and never enough.

Ken roars and Sharon swirls.

Some electronic harmonic whispers, drones, and wavers in the corners of the space, barely holding voice, barely holding synthetics of sound.

Light: penetrates films of flesh, not quite bodies or faces, but lumps
—inebriated metastatic instances.

They all rest on the floor, leaning on walls, at risk of sliding and crashing to the ground.

A portrait of sorts, but not a comfortable one. One that rips at the corners of pleasantries and ignites a deeply rooted sensation that this |will| be you, whether it is cancer, time, or something else.

faced with a discontinuity in Being
Charon waiting
a story you have hidden all of your life
finite yet forever
nested deep in our bodies.
It isn't about death, it is about life, *unfolding in expected ways,*
spontaneous, SUFFERING
vital and rich
not something we want to step out onto.

Illness ends worlds. It is a thin place, between this world and the next. But that is just the world as we know it.
I have been there, maybe you have as well.

pain but maybe an opening. a portal, transformation into a thin place
immediate connection
full of life and living love
reconciliation

endure
or let go.

experience sense sensations come to Know through
suffering

your limits
your body
mind
loves
wounds
conceal
unconceal

origin.

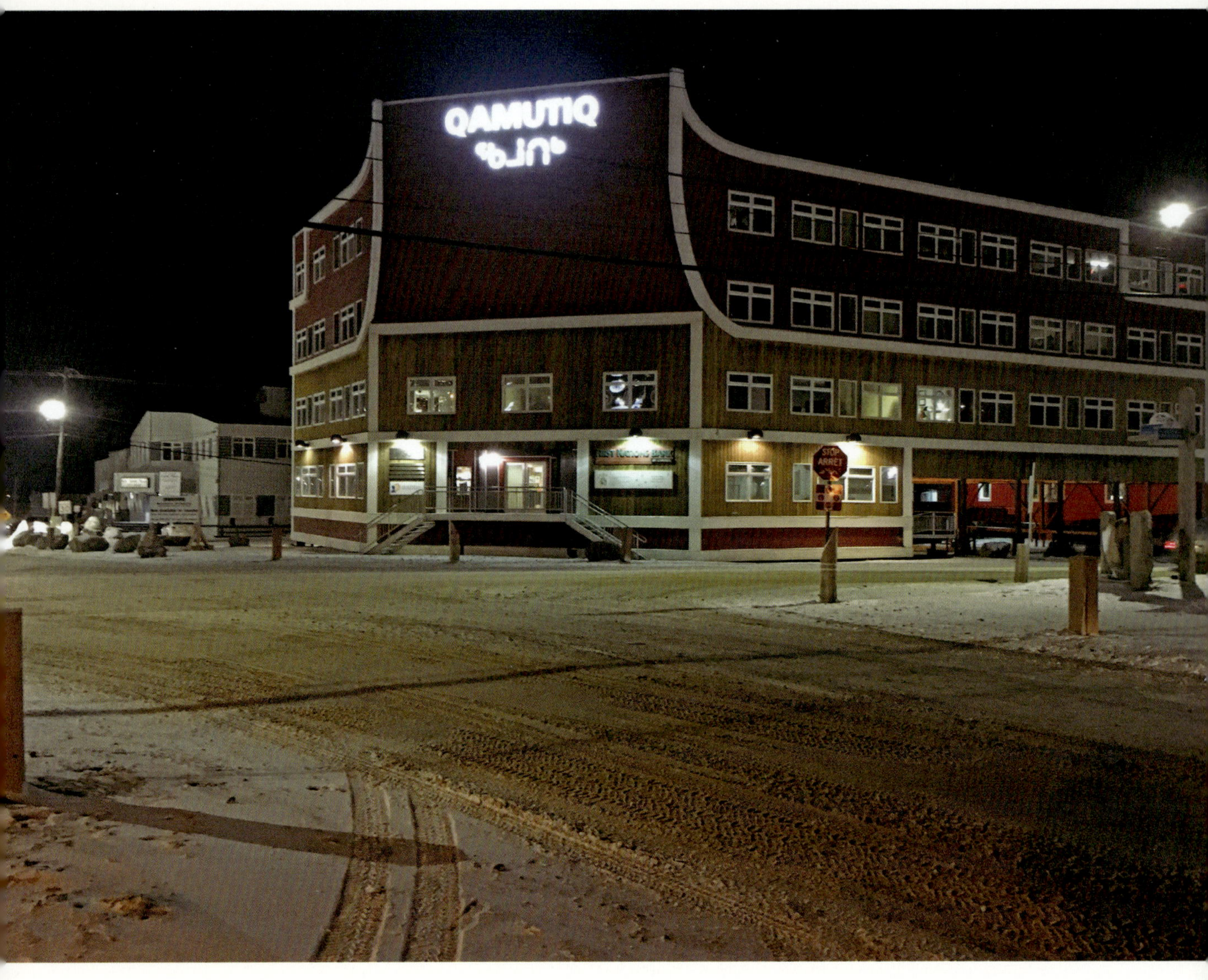

The intersection at Federal Road and Niaqunngusiariaq in Iqaluit.

breathe in breathe out

I slide back behind my eyes, pack on my winter gear, and step outside. Wind pierces this new coat and fur hood. This is a different kind of cold. I look to my right, down the snowy path with the bay pressing on me. Nowhere to go, nowhere to be, I walk straight ahead.

I come to an intersection.

Federal Road and Niaqunngusiariaq.

Government buildings on three corners. Names in Inuktitut. Glyphs to welcome Being.

Ahead, up a hill, full of houses, submarines, and weather stations.

To the left, a small road with speckled buildings. Another hotel and a restaurant in it. The rest disappears into the mist, maybe into a dream.

To the right, a long road full of life and living. I walk down that.

Businesses with colourful, bursting paintings, soapstone, beading, seal skin clothing.

Supermarket.

Tim Hortons.

Red-eye. In need of coffee. Night.

I'll have a large double-double.

She hands me an empty cup.

Okay.

I turn around and see a self-serve counter. I fill it up, use the machine that measures out two sugars and two creams. Tastes just right. Warm.

I walk into the supermarket. I forgot my toiletries: new toothbrush, toothpaste, deodorant, and hair product. One hundred dollars.

Night of black clouds. Limited light pollution. The street is lit but the darkness hangs like a veil. Wind colder and my face aches.

I get back to my hotel and drop off my toiletries. I'll check out the conference taking place in Iqaluit's high school. Fitting home for hope as life and death hang in every corner.

///////////
\\\\\\\\\\\

Earlier, in late August, I am in my supervisor's office. A moment before I had successfully transferred into the PhD program in psychiatry. My co-supervisor, vision-seeker in his heart, Andy Greenshaw, looks up from his phone and says

want to go to Iqaluit?

Embarrassed, I couldn't quite summon up what an "Iqaluit" was.

breathe in
breathe out

Moments ago, I was told I'm here for a journey. I say yes, leave the room, and Google Iqaluit. Right, I remember learning about that in grade school in the late '90s when Nunavut was established. A new Territory.

I go back in.

He says: I can help fund it. It's a conference on suicide. You should present.

That voice in my mind: what do I know about suicide beyond standing on the razor's edge looking down?

He introduces me to the conference organizer.

I write a proposal to give a talk on narrating suicide. Earlier in the year, I wrote a scene in a short film about my suicide, told by an adult Elliot. Maybe I could talk about writing that,,, about hoping that she never has to say those words.

Two weeks later: accepted.

A two-hour workshop.

TWO HOURS.

I thought back to the image theatre workshop for the head and neck cancer group last year. I can't do that.

breathe in breathe out

sure. let's see what I can do

;;;

In October, I take part in another image theatre workshop. I watch David Diamond, theatre director and healer.

How he moves.

How he talks.

How he holds a room.

But this is his job. He wrote a book on it.

On the plane ride, I decide to run a photovoice workshop. Everyone goes around the school and reflects on suicide by taking pictures, framing off the everyday, elevating it by noticing, pausing, sensing, and recording, then we come back and narrate the images: collectively emerging themes. I think I can do that. I think it will fill up two hours.

My awareness returns to my body and I walk to the lobby to catch a cab. I hear a trio of people talking about going to the conference. Maybe we could share a ride. I ask them if I can join them.

sure.

The cab driver asks for seven dollars from each of us. No splitting fairs here.

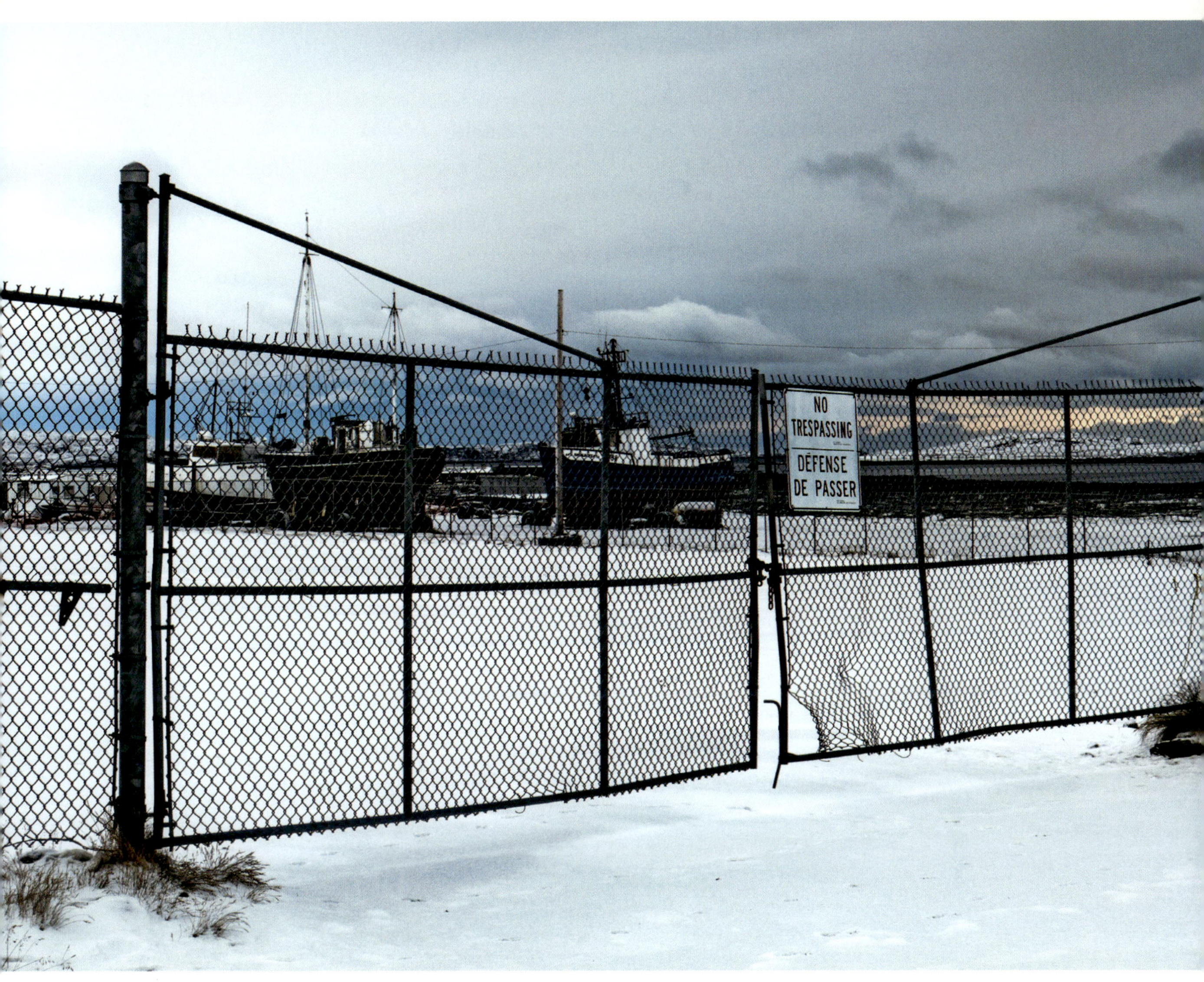

The shipyard on the bay.

We introduce ourselves to each other, all artists running arts-based workshops. They are part of an Indigenous collective based out of Vancouver called Imagi'NATION. As we drove through the darkness, I felt incredible kinship with these new friends in the land beyond the land. *Four connections made, four nodes reflecting each other, radiating up past the black clouded sky, into the hidden Northern Lights, out in hope.*

Late September 2015: a bit over a month into what would become a PhD that I have no idea how I found myself in. Some kind of voice saying:

walk down this trail.

Okay

Pamela Brett-MacLean: Professor, Department of Psychiatry, University of Alberta.

Someone that sees things others don't.

Feels intensely.

Giving and giving.

A guide through the night fog.

Friend. Doctoral supervisor.

Brad, you should come see this image theatre workshop with David Diamond.

A few months before

Sean Caulfield: Centennial Professor, Department of Art and Design, University of Alberta. Visionary artist. Goes into the depths and makes form from no form. Prints from the abyss. Generous.

Minn Yoon: Professor, School of Dentistry, University of Alberta. Stepping into the unknown. Guided by some kind of light. Caring.

These three invite me to be part of a project on head and neck cancer and art. Trying to uncover something, anything about the experience of cancer.

Cancer

a mother at the farm

kids from school: dads

grandma

uncle

aunt

maybe me   feeling for a lump

I have no projects on the go. This is why I start the doctorate. I need something, anything to get going again.

sure

Early morning. I wasn't a morning person yet.

Elevator to the top floor of the School of Business at the University of Alberta.

I enter the room and it is immediately other.

The air carries a sense of bodies, bodies I'm not yet familiar with.

The room's acoustics hang at a low decibel,

growling.

Transfixed: a man reaches for a hole in his neck and a deep sound barks forth. Penetrates my body. Roots me in A BODY. The moment to moment changing body, flux, hoping everything keeps combining and recombining, fighting the gnawing of time and entropy, just as all life on this planet has been trying to.

Where am I?

I don't yet understand it, but I pass through a portal. Sure my eyes and ears are taking this all in, but, without my control, I start to affectively sense this space. My body fills with sensations I have never felt before.

I sit down. Scars, stomas, and sounds of bodies.

I slip

young: maybe ten

farm

a memory or dream not sure of the order

just blasting images and sensations

running up my spine

there was everything

—children parents animals crops warm yellow air standing

stark against the

never-ending blue prairie sky

we were all in the house the mother making us sandwiches

but something was about to happen.

all at once

the mother's funeral my first funeral I sense that this is significant, my

second experience

of something sacred

CANCER, whatever that means

to a child

Twenty years old: I see, again, how quickly cancer can take.

Driving home from the hospital I feel my abdomen. I feel something foreign in me.

I go to the doctor, tests, but only a

spectre in the periphery.

A belch, then a gasp out of a throat stoma collapses me into the room. New sounds: constant. I look to my side and see a woman with a scar line from her lip to the bottom of her throat. When she speaks I felt the absence of her tongue. I couldn't make out the words.

I slope down in my chair.

breathe in

breathe

out in out

I open my awareness (before I even know what that means) and sense the evolving sensations rushing through my conscious experience and a body: the root of the root.

<<< Flash forward to May 2018: Chicago's International Museum for Surgical Sciences. *FLUX: Head and Neck Cancer* exhibition. Today, the symposium. My turn. After reading the sentence above, I say:

I am tremendously uncomfortable, but I also realize that I am seeing something most people don't see—hidden people.

The head and neck cancer patients are in the crowd. I hope I don't wound them with that line. But that is the sensation.

After I finish, a patient gets up and says she *does* feel like a hidden person.

She says:

thank you for recognizing that.

but

after this year   and   year
exhibition   and exhibition
surgery   and treatment
friend   seen,
the project ,   art   I don't feel that way anymore.

(Holy angel!
She is radiating like a solar flare. She is seen!
Worlded,   validated
she is witnessed. she is not alone.) >>>

Back in the Business School of 2015, we are introduced to the project:

Artists, head and neck cancer patients, their families, researchers, and clinicians will spend the next two days unveiling something, anything, that we can investigate through art over the next year.

I open to this experience.

As the day continues, there is a sense of reverence for what these people, these family members, have endured. It hangs like a viscous affect, sticking to me, pulling into my throat, choking me.

David Diamond:

can someone get up and make a shape with their body?

No movement.

Okay.

I get up and make a gesture with my arms.

David:

can someone else make a shape with him?

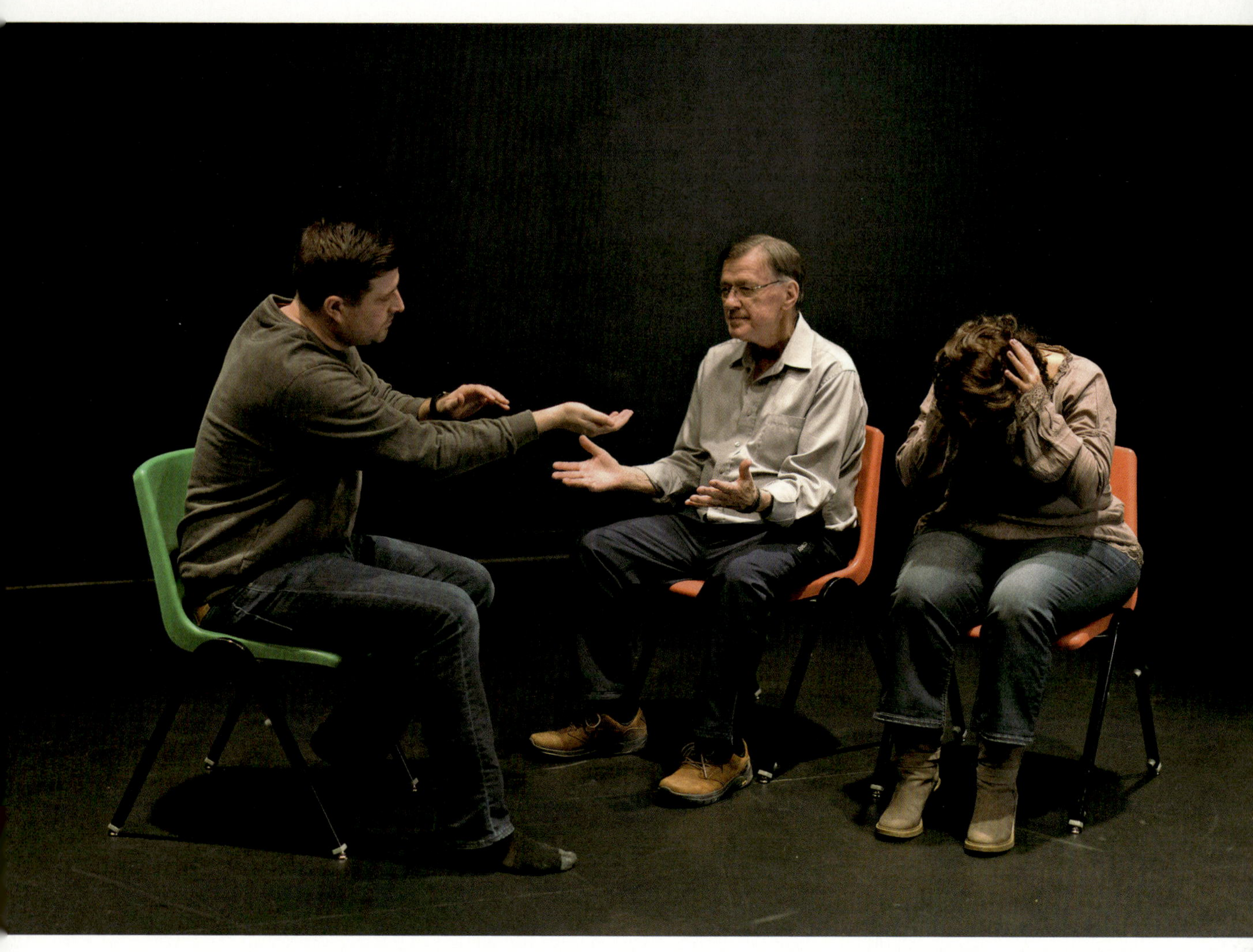

Head and neck cancer image theatre workshop, October 2015, University of Alberta.

Image after image, there were stories of struggle, of surviving, of battles, and of hope—full of philosopher Susan Sontag's war metaphors, the ones she describes as she fights breast cancer. These are the kinds of metaphors we see on TV, in movies, in the news, and in pamphlets for charity drives.

Soon, our bodies overlap, tissue reaching across the mental void, connecting, overlapping, binding: telling larger, longer stories I don't understand intellectually, but ones that unmoor my soul. At the time, I story these sensations as discomfort, but writing this now I don't story them that way anymore. It's love. But not the side of love that bursts from your heart as you start falling.

no

the other side.

This is the painful outer love of connection—*we are all in it together. Losing distinctions where there always were none, between ~~you~~ and ~~me~~ or rolling abyss, falling, growing closer,*

awakening, losing the dream,

merging,

ecstasy, the flow of becoming, and all of everything.

I get home and I am restless. Not something a pill or bourbon could fix, but one that needs form.

I appropriate images, digitally stack them, ravage them, cut them. Violence

ripping | disintegrating | bleeding faces—one

pain

It is happening.

The thing we are always hiding from

and,

I'm hiding from gamma-ray bursts from far off galaxies.

I print the images, put them in these dental lightboxes I had collected two years before.

I turn them on and flick off the lights.

No one would ever want to see this.

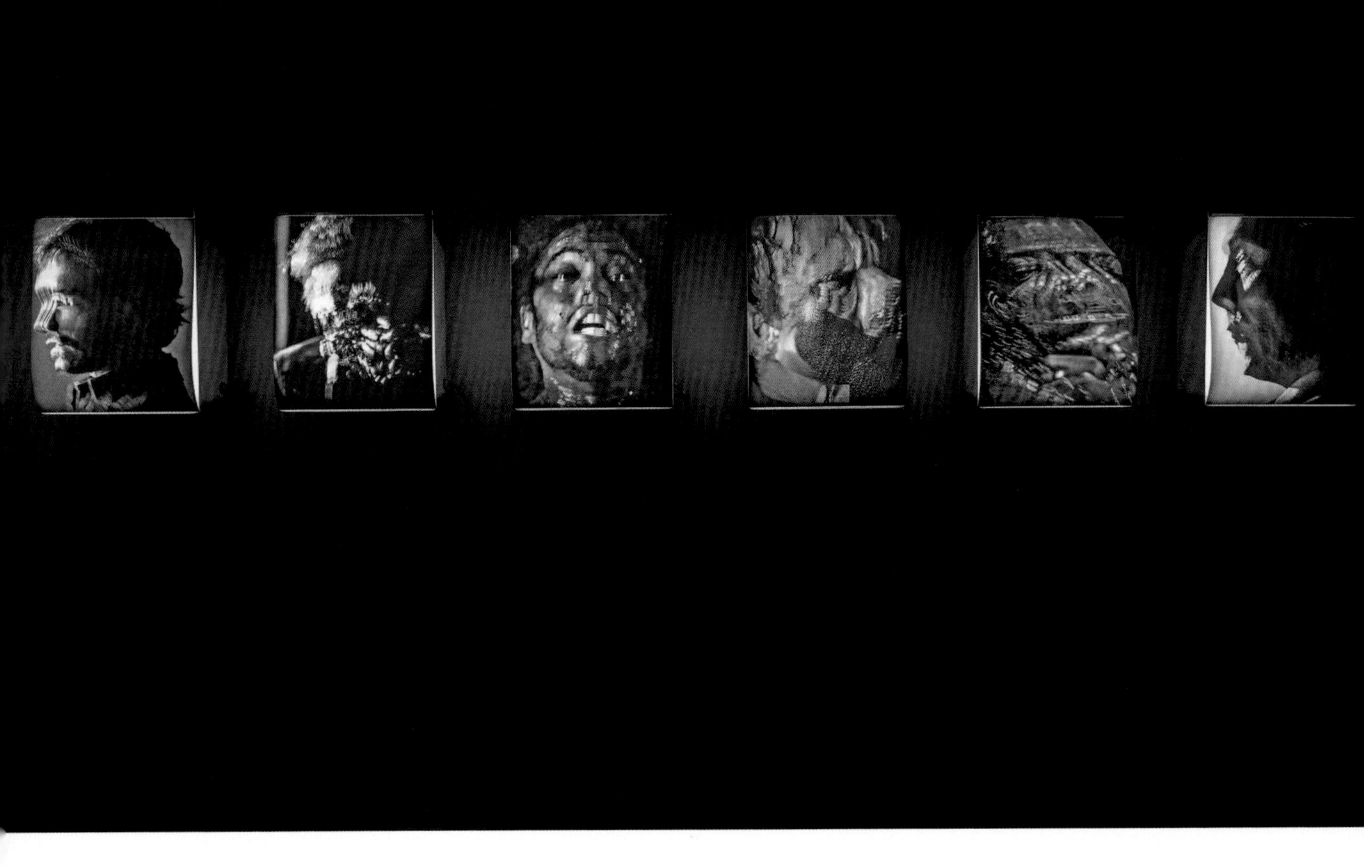

Waiting Room, 2015.
Initial response to the image theatre workshop in October 2015, University of Alberta.

A RESEARCH MEETING

February 2016: very official research meeting at the University of Alberta. Cancer is as serious as it gets. Much more important people are talking about important things and I gaze out the window with no view other than a grey hallway.

We are doing important stuff is what I hear.

Brad.

My mind collapses the wave function of daydreaming, a portal into Otherworlds, and crashes into my body, looking out these eyes. Mouth begins to move. I say ::

I was inspired by our image theatre workshop and made an artwork in response.

I show them the six lightbox image.

Horror

and repulsion

by the violent disfiguration.

They believe this would hurt the patient participants.

  No one should see these images.

There is a bit of back and forth about what art has to offer this project.

I slip back into a daydream, sensing the sensations that are coursing through my body and mind, drifting down

and down.

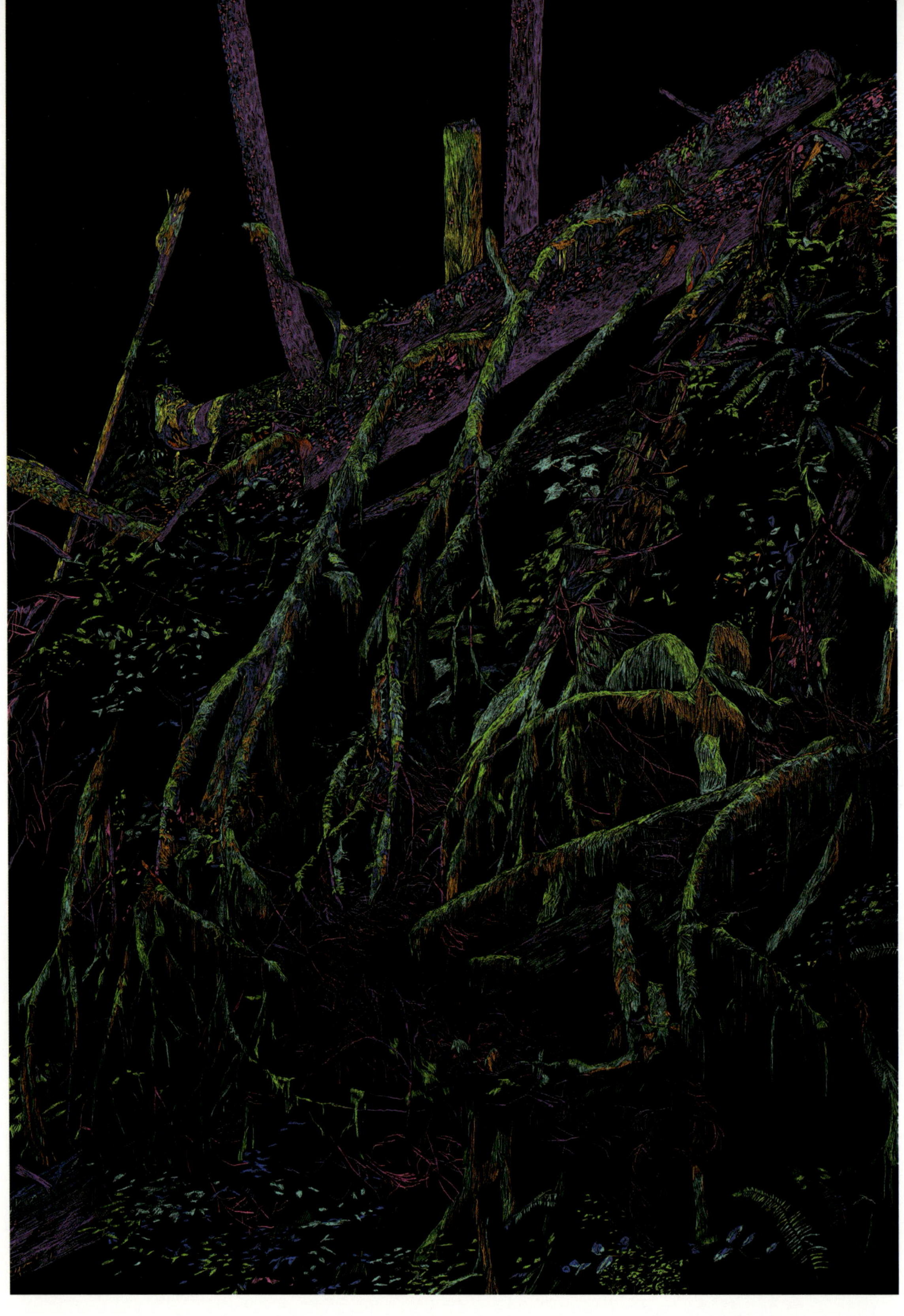

Avatar's Dream #3, 2021.
Digital drawing.

I am speaking as an artist.

A philosopher, priest, mystic, or a banker might have different ideas.

Being is ineffable.

Like the Tao: a description is not absolute Being.

A relationship with the abyss unconceals Being, reorients us into the open. *To be in the open is to be with and within Being—flowing and becoming.* The abyss is a teacher; with awe, terror, and love, it teaches you to remove your Self, to become a mirror that holds onto nothing, a column of air that flows as it becomes—it cannot be held, a distinct moment or thing, but is simply flow from moment to moment, breath to breath, being to being that we *are*.

Being before Being is to be nobody: merging. Oneness with infinite parts. One becomes many to come to Know itself.

A gradient.

As a being, you are broken into parts to come to Know Being, to understand what it is to be one.

Becoming

Enlightenment

Individuation

Self-Actualization

Being is the warmth that shelters when you lose the properties of being a
Self,
a consciousness and unconsciousness,
a human separate from life,
a human in an environment,
with the cosmos radiating out-there,
life
death,
and sensation and hallucination radiating in-here.

It orients you to Be. It teaches you how to live, lifting the burden, the suffering of being a being thrust into the porousness of life.

So perfect incarnation.

Being is a state of conscious awareness outside of and beyond the waking consciousness, the one that tells you story after story, the layers of story laying like a trap, a trap that keeps you from bathing in the open.

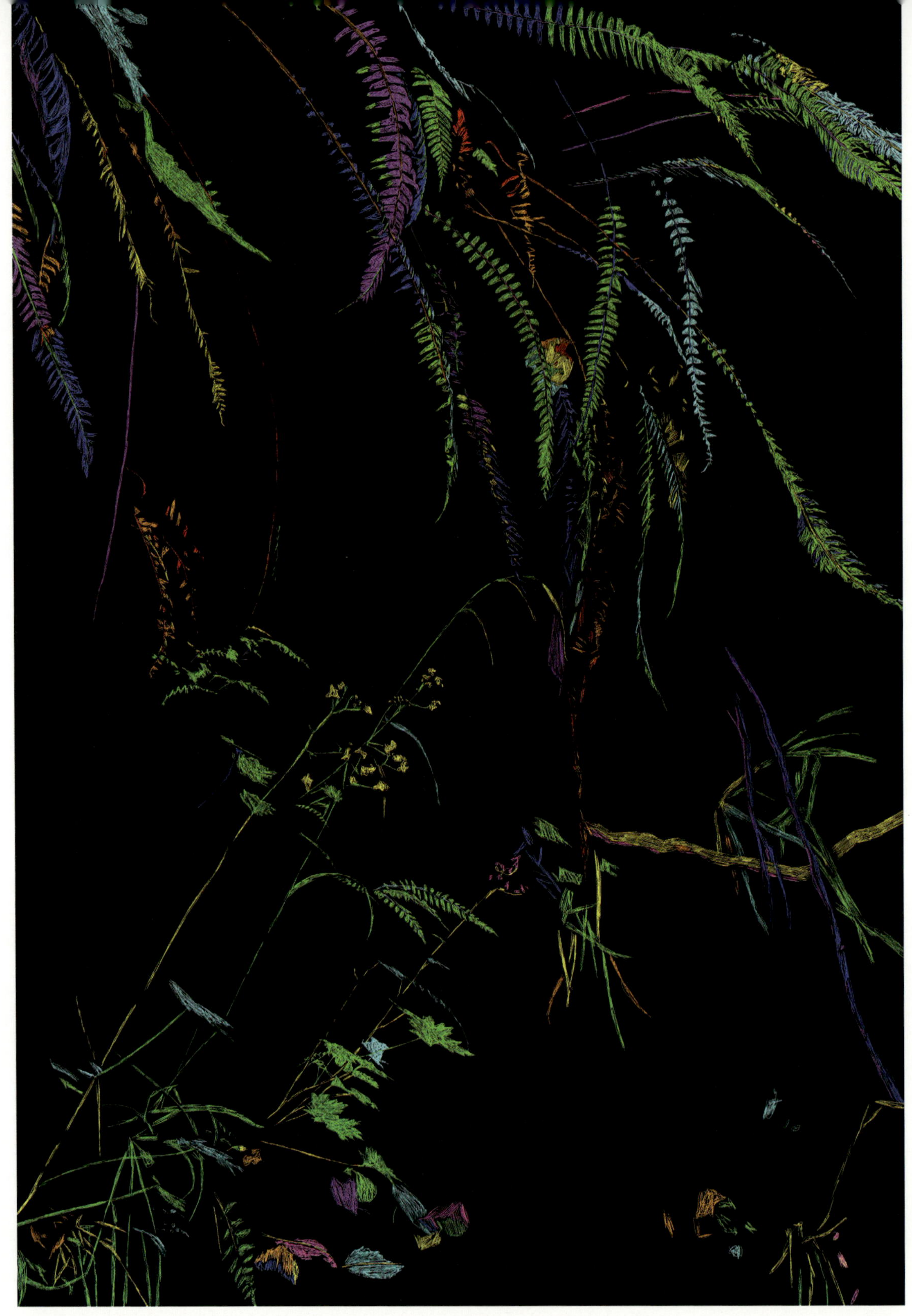

Avatar's Dream #2, 2021.
Digital drawing.

Entropy is the unravelling of everything to disorder, it gives us the arrow of time from the Big Bang onwards, as the universe unfolds from perfection—one, a pure singularity—to less and less order: the forward march of time.

Life is the unfolding process that lowers entropy to a miracle. Life is constantly unstitching and unravelling. Living is the process of healing the pull of entropy.

To keep life expressing we heal, the moment to moment miracle of living, holding together the breath to breath becoming with and within Being.

Healing is Life.

To heal, leave the grips of holding onto a Self
and enter into a state of becoming,   where one is in flux, falling, merging, and opening to the inner and outer universe. To stay in a state of becoming one must find a Charon that bypasses the Self where one enters into the clearing of the open, a pure space of experience where one confronts other orientations to Being. These orientations open or conceal the possibility of the flow of experience from moment to moment,
being to being,
either alleviating suffering or enhancing it—personally, collectively, spiritually.

Everyone needs to heal. We have to heal the
ceasure
that happened from incarnation, where we lost our oneness with
our   consciousness,
our   body,
our   experience,
our   Mother, Earth
our   World
—slowly forming a Self in the most evolutionarily recent parts of the brain:
the Default-Mode Network.

Developing the Self that started making containers with an inside and outside, separation, distinctions where there is no distinction. This is oneness becoming many. We do this to come to Know ourselves. Healing is dissolving this ceasure, the Self, the ego, turning off the Default-Mode Network, getting outside of stories. To do this we fall into the abyss, gaze into its radiance and splendour, and merge. This is the healing journey.

Creative practice is a crucial way by which we enter into the open. Sometimes you are creating something that looks like art, sometimes not.

Indra insists for me to look closer:

I look up and see the forest canopy silhouette, cutting out the night sky:

moon, stars, heaven.

I see the web of the mind, fashioned just right

to catch the universe. Collect majesty.

Collect the consciousness of the conscious universe.

I am in a forest in the Pacific Northwest

and a mist is collecting on a web, forming perfect droplets.

I move closer.

I see myself wrapping around a droplet with the forest,

moon, and

heaven

fused as one on the

surface.

I look closer.

I see all the droplets

along the web, with all

their reflections,

reflecting in the droplet

as well. And all of

everything in each

droplet. I am worlding

the droplet in place

and the droplet is

worlding me and all of

everything in our place.

I look back to the moon reflecting the illumination of the sun warming some far off land, and from 384,400 km away it is worlding me in foot and I am worlding it in its gravity well.

I feel further to the light from the Cosmic Microwave Background shining the birth of a new universe. It worlds me and I world the beginning of time.

The universe is witnessing itself.

Art is a web I fashion, that catches my inner universe. A mist in a forest of the mind collects on it and reflects me in its droplets. I am seen. I am witnessed.

I am witnessing myself.

Self-showing. Knowing.

Sometimes you create art, sometimes not. Then, sometimes, you are creating yourself—to erect and dissolve You, to

Become,

to Heal.

On November 11, 2017, sitting on a rooftop in Arizona I write that I feel the world in pain. Today, June 3, 2020, two and a half months into the COVID-19 pandemic lockdown and nine days into the George Floyd protests I also feel the world in pain. Sitting in the relative comfort of a small suburb in Canada I simply open myself to that pain. I meditate on this pain as I sit outside feeling the warmth of the sun and the chilled everywhere wind. I feel sadness, I feel anger, I long for justice, part of me wants to see it burn, reborn from the ashes, another part of me simply wants to cry. I should cry.

I should cry, but the dose of antipsychotics I'm on acts like a dam. Damn.

Then I look to the future, maybe to the next wave of COVID in the fall, and I feel scared, filling with uncertainty. My friend aAron Munson tells me that the apocalypse is a time of revelation that can only be known in its unfolding. So I meditate on this.

I sit on the grass, feeling the earth below me, the grass that tickles and itches a bit,
I listen to the buzzing of insects,
hear the wind filled with ancestors and change,
watch my breath,
in and out,
I take in the vibrant orange and pink visual field behind my eyelids,
the photons exploding out of nuclear fusion at the centre of the sun,
travelling eight minutes through the void,
to pierce my eyelids,
illuminate my rods and cones,
radiate in my synaptic clefts,
and burst sensation into the abyss of consciousness,
pressing against thoughts that want to run run run,
and I take in the beauty of that colour,
the passing of time,
how I am mixing with the sun,   mixing with the air,
mixing with the birch tree's pollen
that itches my nose
and I rocket my mind into the ground,   through the soil,   the clay,   the granite,
the molten core,   out the back of the Earth,   out to space,   past the moon,
and out of mind.

Twenty-five hundred years ago a being sits under a Bodhi tree and realizes that suffering is universal. Suffering is the cause to bring about its end. Suffering is part of the dipole of Being, along with joy, bliss, or any other positive impression, expression. Both joy and suffering push us to Know ourselves, through their conflict, through their strife. It is only through strife that Knowing can be won—the unconcealment of Being. And so I meditate on this.

I feel myself in a continuum of beings, spontaneous life, unfolding,
expressing its essence:
I see an eagle gliding on currents never beating its wings,
a flower peeling itself from the ground and bathing the world in colour and dying in the
first freeze,
the black hole's Being impressing its gravity well on my Being,
dying, then transformation,
being to being,
to forming form to express the depths of no-form,
visionary art,
death,
creating a Self,
boundaries and boxes with insides and outsides,
the suffering of being trapped or locked looking in from the outside,
concealing Being,
then birth and death and rebirth.

Then I sense the collecting Charons across time as I create outside of mind. As I fall into visions. Or become consumed by mania as the 100-mile tidal wave of Being obliterates my Self. Or evaporating the doors of perception with psychedelics that could be the tipping point for 7.8 billion revolutions. Or the meditation on moment to moment, breath to breath alignment of Being, unconcealing, to become a mirror that holds nothing, and I become nothing and no one,
one.

I sense back into my body and feel the hydrogen glow of the sun and its warmth, giving, and Being and thinking about George Floyd and if my daughter will go back to school next year, and the weight of gravity in my chest as the universe within is collapsing into the abyss, and I sit with that and let the Charon of meditation take me past the event horizon and I rest on suffering.

I am writing this to be with suffering. To sense it, to feel it course through my body, blister my mind, feeling for a rupture, a haemorrhage. Maybe I will cry.

I want to tell you a story, or a series of stories, about some experiences of *everything* I have.

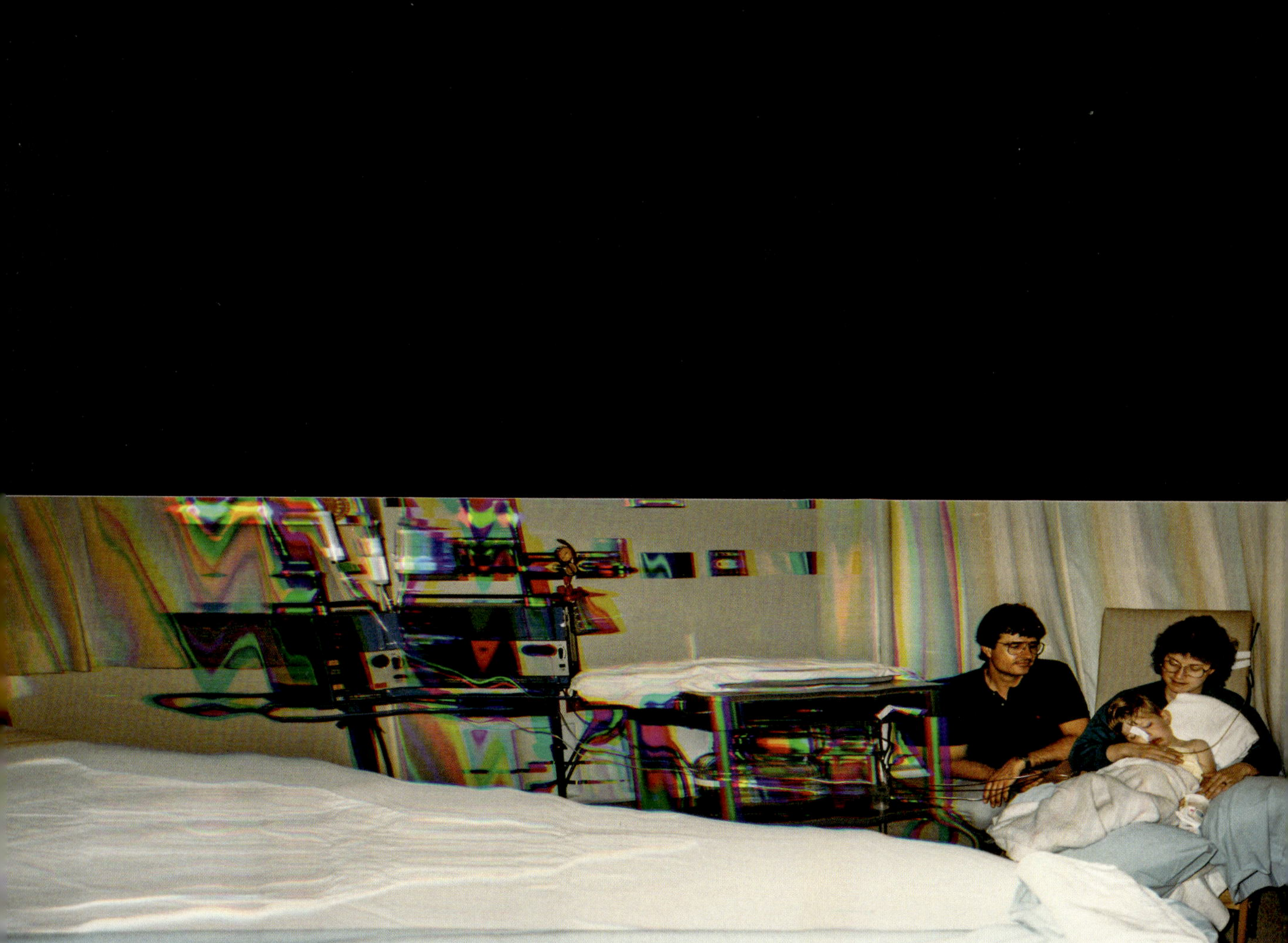

The University Hospital
Edmonton, Alberta, 1987.
My Grandpa Necyk was
a photographer. He took
this photograph.

1987

I have strong parents
love
but I was a sick kid error in my intestines malformed
no nerves.

I had lots of surgeries
taking parts of me out putting plastic in
taking that out
then six metal stitches leaving me partly open to not trap
an infection
incredibly rare disease
I was sick from day one, but my mom fought for me
doctors' offices
waiting rooms
tests, pain
but my mom never gave up.
I remember the surgery. Not with visions or sound, but a deep hunger
no food for ten days as my intestines grew back together.

I remember my hands a thickness to them a weight a uselessness.
They tape oven mitts on me. My mom says it was so I couldn't pull out all the
tubes running into me.
I spent the next ten years with side effects and pain growing around this pain.

I am writing this to be with that pain, sense this suffering, trying to heal from
something so long ago it feels like a dream.

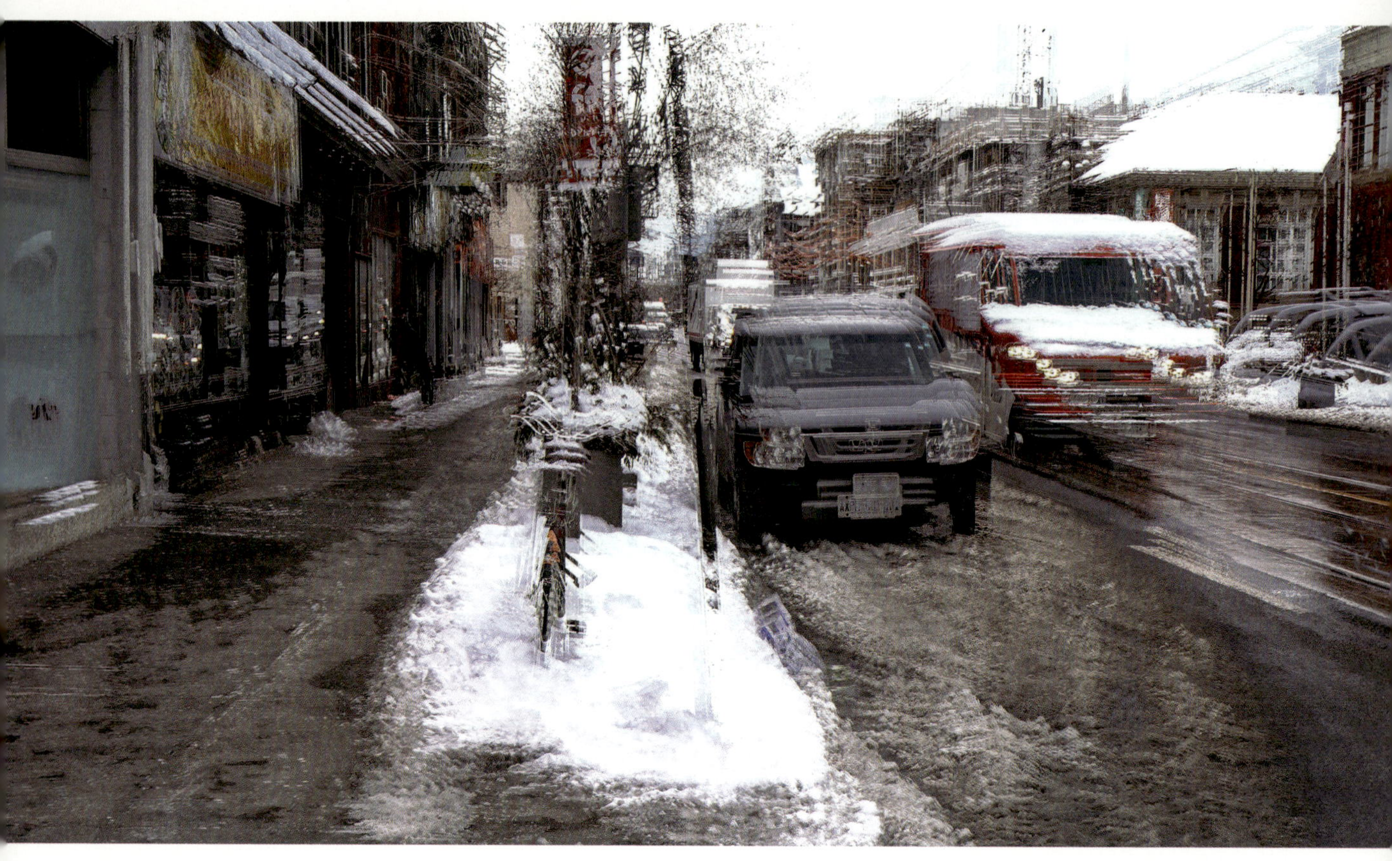

Looking down Queen Street in Toronto towards the Centre for Addiction and Mental Health (CAMH), February 2017.

THE CENTRE FOR ADDICTION AND MENTAL HEALTH, TORONTO, ONTARIO

February 8, 2017:

Red-eye to Toronto. Take my mood stabilizer, antipsychotic, anti-anxiety, and sleeping pills on the plane. Sleep: three hours. Not enough to dissolve these pills from concealing my Being.

Uber from the airport. Sixty dollars.

The Drake Hotel. Toronto famous. Designer room. Beautiful.

6 a.m.

Collapse on the bed. Meeting at 8:30 a.m.

10 a.m. Wake up, get in fresh clothes and spill onto Queen Street. Blurry, cold, but not like Edmonton. The front desk says the hospital is not a long walk.

Lots of construction, traffic. City noise. The cold air off Lake Ontario is waking me up.

10 minutes.

Large sign: Centre for Addiction and Mental Health. CAMH. Pronounced Cam-H.

Many buildings. I don't know which one to go in. One says: Education. I enter, wander down a hall, door, another hall, then, luck, the office I was directed to.

I give my name. They call my contact in the Youth with Concurrent Addiction Unit.

They take my picture, give me a badge, a bunch of keys, and an email address.

I first hear about CAMH through Candace, years before.

This is the largest psychiatric treatment and research hospital in Canada.

June 2016: after finishing as the artist-in-residence at the University Hospital in Edmonton working with transplant patients, I thought I could do another. I put together a package and gave it to Candace's aunt who volunteers at CAMH.

One person to the next.

Phone call: Dr. Ivan Silver, psychiatrist, VP Education at CAMH. Open heart. The kind of psychiatrist I dreamed of having.

What is this all about?

I'm a doctoral student in psychiatry looking at the lived experience of mental illness and recovery. I would like to do some fieldwork at CAMH. Co-create art with patients. Like I did with the transplant patients and was starting to with the head and neck cancer patients.

The word co-create really resonates with people—*we are in it together.*

He says:

okay.

It takes six months and a bunch of administrative work between the University of Alberta and the University of Toronto, but in February 2017, I was taking the elevator up to the Youth Unit.

Ivan thought it was important I start with the children.

The unit manager uses her keys to open a door, then another door, and then we found our way into the unit. Glass nurses station, like Foucault's panopticon, then a long hallway with all the private rooms. The building was new, not what I expected.

Introduced to some staff, tired eyes, also, my tired eyes.

I forgot to get coffee on my way here.

BANG BOOM BOOM.

The unit manager asked me if I would like to join the patients in the drum circle.

Okay.

She opened the door and BOOM. Large drums tucked between kids legs, hands beating, life breathing.

Volunteer leading: looks past my eyes and gestures to a drum at the side.

I grab it, sit in an open chair and just start drumming.

Instructor sounds sick, but he presses on. Giving new rhythms, breathing force. So many volunteers I would meet. Couldn't imagine recovery without them.

Hours before: red-eye.

BOOM BOOM.

I slip

surface rhythms sheep skin, finger palm
BOOM
look around kids, teenagers
body uncomfortable mind uncomfortable

BOOM

where am I again?
artist PhD pychiatry psychiatric hospital Toronto no sense
am I a patient? yet?

hammering on BOOM BOOM boom

Drifting down and down.
Maybe like sleeping, thought at that time. Now I Know it's something else

fall

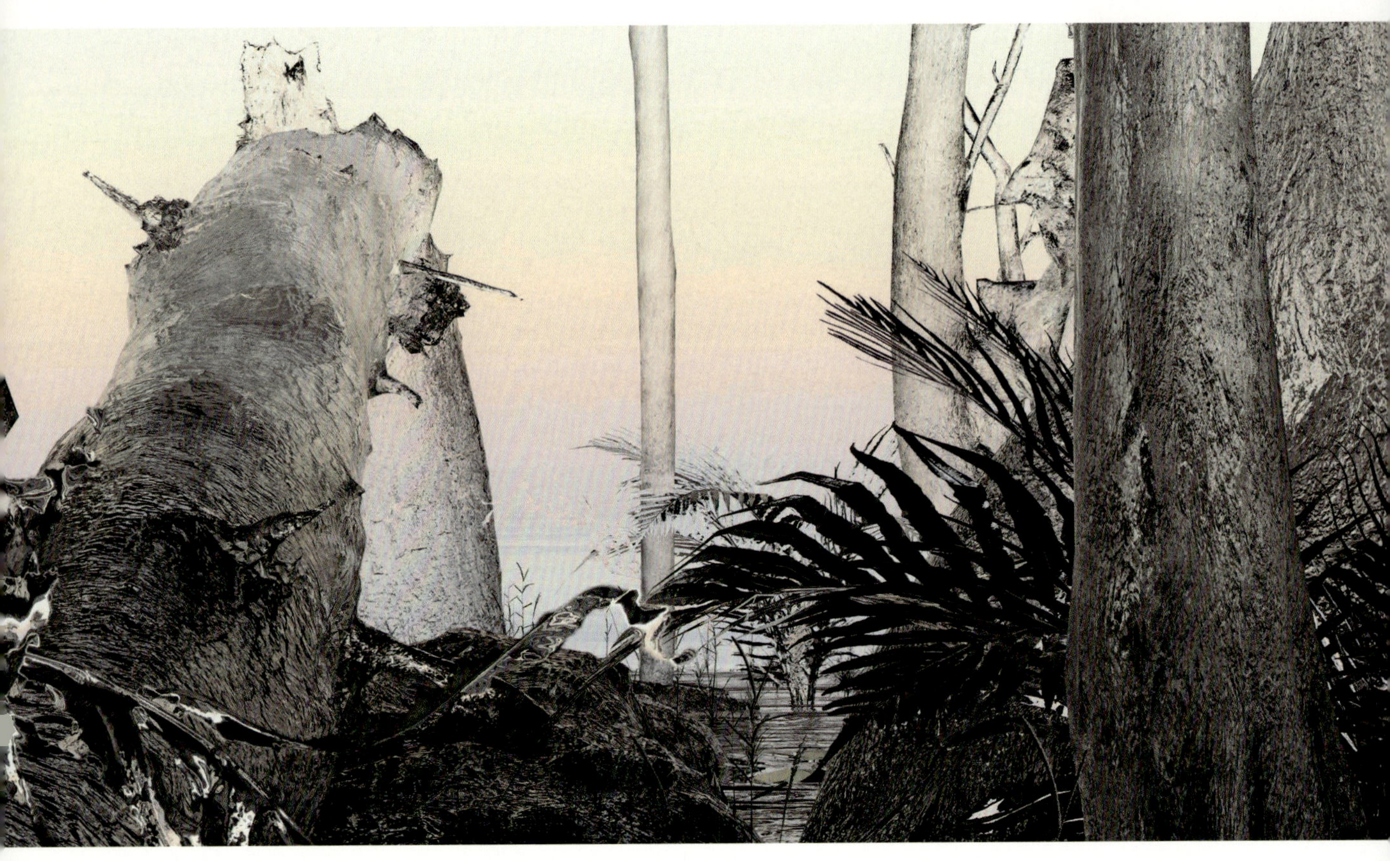

ALL SKY, MIRROR OCEAN, 2021. 6-minute video created with musician Jonathan Kawchuk for MUTEK 2021.

Day seven of ten: CAMH.

I call Candace from my hotel room, in the shower, trying to ground myself in the flow of water: also warmth. Shelter.

We leave the day after I get back from Toronto for Mexico: family vacation.

I am

agitated
crawling
anxious
sad

UNWELL. TAN WALLS. Being with the kids is too difficult.
Trying to stay above water. Mental sky cascading.

I saw my children there.
I see myself as a child there.
I cry, begging to avoid coming to Mexico.
{{{Elliot can stay home with me}}}
Candace says I need to come. It will be good for me.
then: I should take a break from the hospital.

// It matters what matters we use to think other matters with;
it matters what stories we tell to tell other stories with;
it matters what knots knot knots,
what thoughts think thoughts,
what descriptions describe description,
what ties tie ties.
It matters what stories make worlds, what worlds make stories //.
—Donna Haraway, *Staying with the Trouble*

In spring 2017, writing about art in the Anthropocene with Dan, I first learn about stories that are *just big enough* from Donna Haraway. Haraway: philosopher, and a towering figure in my Being. She has been the spark for countless inner revolutions. She weaves and knots, telling me stories of love and hope: reorientation. Stories that aren't too big to climb into or too small to breathe into, but ripping with potential to *do* something—*anything can be better than this*. Attuning to scales, in space and time and, now spirit, the eternal realms of

ecstasy and revelation.

Removing the viewer from projections backwards and forwards and all around, and rooting them to the earth between their toes and the Earth dancing in gravity wells across spacetime. Maybe this can be the start of a billion inner revolutions, reorientations to Being, losing ourselves and becoming one with infinite parts. I don't understand that in 2017, but I am sensing it now.

First, too big, then, too small, perfect, just big enough.

Just right.

In fall 2017, I am reading Haraway and she says: // It matters what stories make worlds, what worlds make stories. // I see threads of hope ebbing and flowing as I breathe that in and out over years like a mantra, in for the next meditation and out across the abyssal expanse between beings and time. The world at my feet and into the sky, the world that warms and shelters, and the world of the cosmos and the world of the micro, nano, atomic, quantum, planck. Yet also, the inner world of revolution towards unfolding and passing into the spirit of becoming.

It matters,

matters of hope.

On New Year's Day in 2018, I lie on an outdoor sofa on the seventh floor of an apartment in Mexico: family vacation. Looking out at the expanse before me, I feel the sun's heat reflecting off the ocean, onto the page, and into mind. Reading the then-unpublished draft of Natalie Loveless's *How to Make Art at the End of the World: A Manifesto for Research-Creation*.

For me, Natalie Loveless is a bodhisattva,
the teacher, thinker, professor
(Illumination! Holy!)
warmth of a mother giving,
Stormshelter.

I tangle with Thomas King's *The Truth about Stories* and with Haraway again, *The Companion Species Manifesto* this time, and I see how artists are storytellers. Sometimes in the linear line of word and breath, and sometimes in the totality of a vision outside of the forward march of time and progress, falling into despair at the aching, slipping sensations of descent, madness, and immortality.

Behold.

Beholden.

Natalie radiates in my Being as she breathes stories that // promise some futures and conceal others. // It's a promise that binds us — *we are in this together* — and one that aids us // to see some things and not others. // Maybe I don't want to see, it's too bright. This is not a desire, but a need. So here I am, writing these words and meditating on Being.

Coming across this quote from Thomas King— // Want a different ethic? Tell a different story // my mind immediately translates it as:

Want a different *world*?

Tell a different story.

With their gestures to the abyss, Loveless, Haraway, and King give me footing to step out, to step forward, to take steps that change my worldline, my worlds both of spacetime and of spirit.

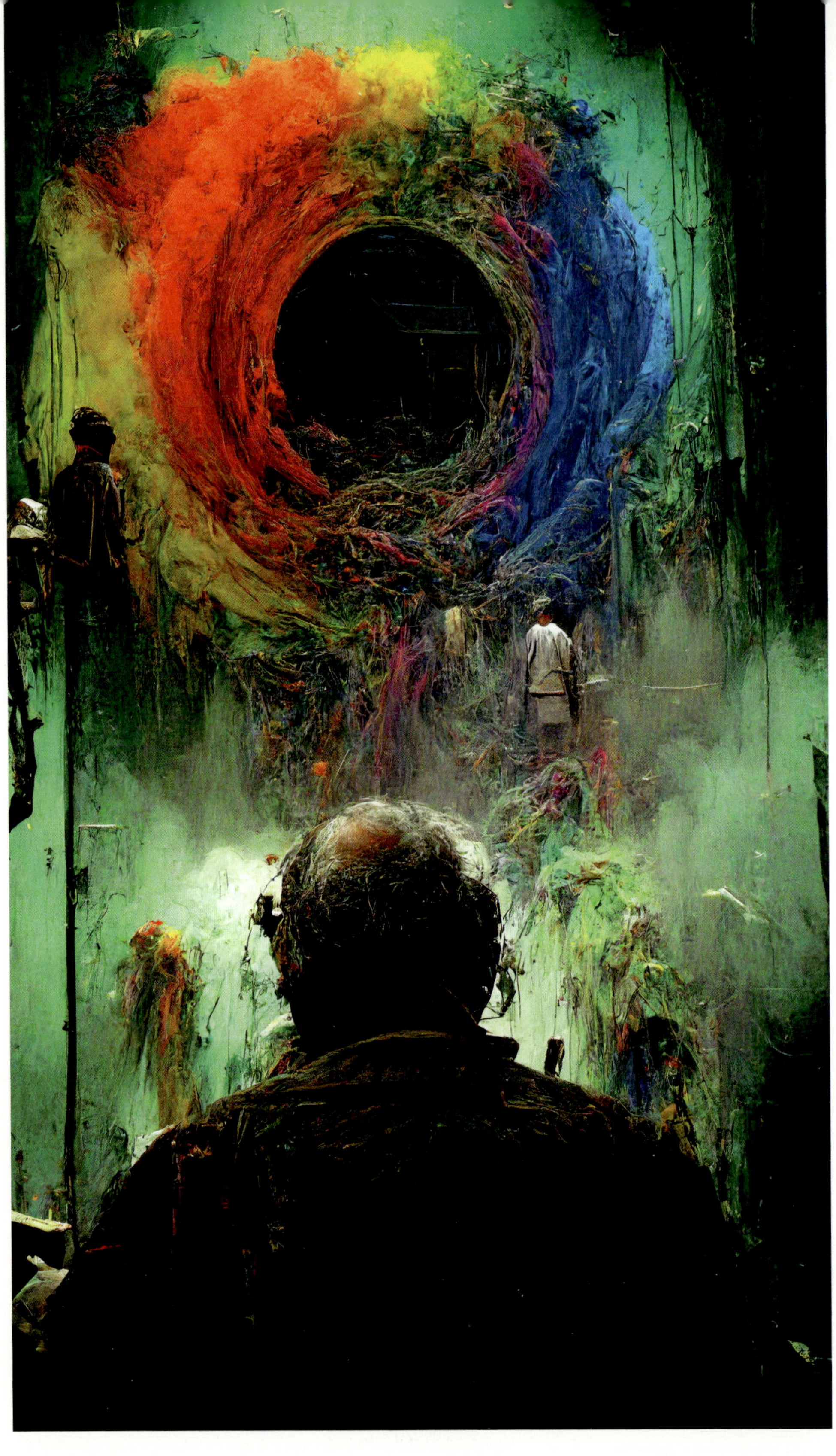

The Birth of a World, 2022. Artificial intelligence generated image.

Giorgio Agamben: philosopher. For me, the great translator. First, biopolitics, now worlding and the open. Giving me a glimpse into spaces I could not reach alone.

In 2011 I read Agamben's *The Open*. It fades like a dream but restructures my mind to unconsciously world worlds—a play with a noun to a verb: generating.

Today, March 29, 2020, on day sixteen of self-isolation waiting for lab results during the COVID-19 pandemic, I reread *The Open* with fresh eyes, a changed mind, and a new world. It resonates from front to back.

A primordial image presents itself in my mind. A world-generating being,
in a clearing, but a closed loop, eyes turned back.
All unto its own.
Looking at the being ;;; wholeness with infinite parts,
but the being is lost to its Self on Indra's Net. !Blind!
then,

ILLUMINATION!

Voice: fall
lose the traps placed all around
fall
event horizon presents
slip
then, the being is no one, in the opening, sifting gradient falling,
then, merging,
one
with infinite connections and reflections.

I feel each being on the Earth and in the cosmos, *like every grain of sand has its own name*, and I experience something I don't understand yet. The open.

Agamben breathes Jakob von Uexküll: biologist writing in the 1920s. Uexküll distinguishes between the *Umgebung*, the world-out-there or the objective world, and the *Umwelt*, an infinite set of perceptual, subjective worlds of each being, *each grain of sand*, that interacts with the *Umgebung* through a unique set of perceptions: carriers of significance. Each species has its own set of perceptions crucial for survival. The being worlds its world with these perceptions, unique to each being. *It promises some worlds and conceals others. You see some things and not others.*

Donald Hoffman, contemporary cognitive psychologist, Professor, University of California Irvine, revolutionary; builds on these perceptual worlds, saying we do not world anything from the world-out-there but inhabit a personal world, a world shaped by the pressures of evolution that relies on efficiency over accuracy. Our perceptual world is a hallucination that resembles nothing out-there, hidden behind the veil of senses, of perception, of worlding. Central to his exploration is the idea:

consciousness is fundamental. Everything is conscious.

Forget matter begetting consciousness; forever butting our heads: *the hard problem of consciousness.*

No.

Consciousness begets everything. Quantum mechanics, general relativity, and, to dream and dream and dream, the Theory of Everything will fall out of Hoffman and his team's conscious agent equations. Math is the study of consciousness, feeling out its folds and fissures. They are mapping the inner and outer universe simultaneously: one.

He continues

Our world is our own hallucination yet we have portals to merge with others. We are pretty good at opening portals to other humans, less so with, say, a cat, less with an ant (we could hardly imagine that world), and there is no portal to a rock's world (but that does not exclude the possibility of that rock's world). Can you imagine a portal to the abyss?

A whirlpool is a portal. So is a black hole. They are portals with event horizons. You can't go back to the way things were after crossing over, crossing that horizon.

The |thin place| between this realm and the next.

Visionary artists are thin places, giving birth to event horizons.

Their artworks are portals that begin the birth of a new universe. A new world to inhabit and sense.

It's scary. I know. You don't have to fall. But no matter what, you will, someday:

death.

Visionary art ferries you across, elicits the sensation of sensations.

Maybe, these stories will help you come to the edge and glimpse. See the raging primordial ocean, the circling galaxy around the supermassive blackhole. Feel its pull. Are you afraid of heights? Only perhaps because part of you simply, plainly, wants to fall.

breathe in, breathe out

We will get there together.

✳ In July 2020, I move to Vancouver Island and am looking out at the expanse of ocean and Mt. Baker behind the bluing haze of coastal humidity. It feels so alive, with or without witness, but here I am witnessing it,

or so it feels.

I feel the ocean breeze cool my skin, then an eagle flies above me, now the pressing of the hot hot sun. I sit on a rock near the edge of a small mountain, gazing into the expanse before me and I feel all the accumulated heat of the day radiating off the rock pushing upwards on my body. So hot I move my feet to rest on some small plants that don't hold the heat and I meditate. I came here for this moment. 13.8 billion years of movement and I am here worlding this experience:

alignment.

There is something out there, peaking through the doors of perception, but I know it isn't anything like this experience. But that doesn't make this experience, these sensations, this world any less perfect. I don't think I need to experience the quantum field or dark matter or gamma rays to heal, to Be. *Cosmic and genomic evolution gave me all I need.* Instead, this gradient as the ocean moves to sky and the sky moves through all the blues I could ever hope for is what all these 13.8 billion years have been working towards.

So perfect is incarnation.

Sensing Being through a body and mind full of turbulence and uncertainty, emotions and pain, but also bliss and love. Coming to Know myself through spontaneous life, the essence of flow, and

holy! everything.

Worlding this sacred hallucination within Being.

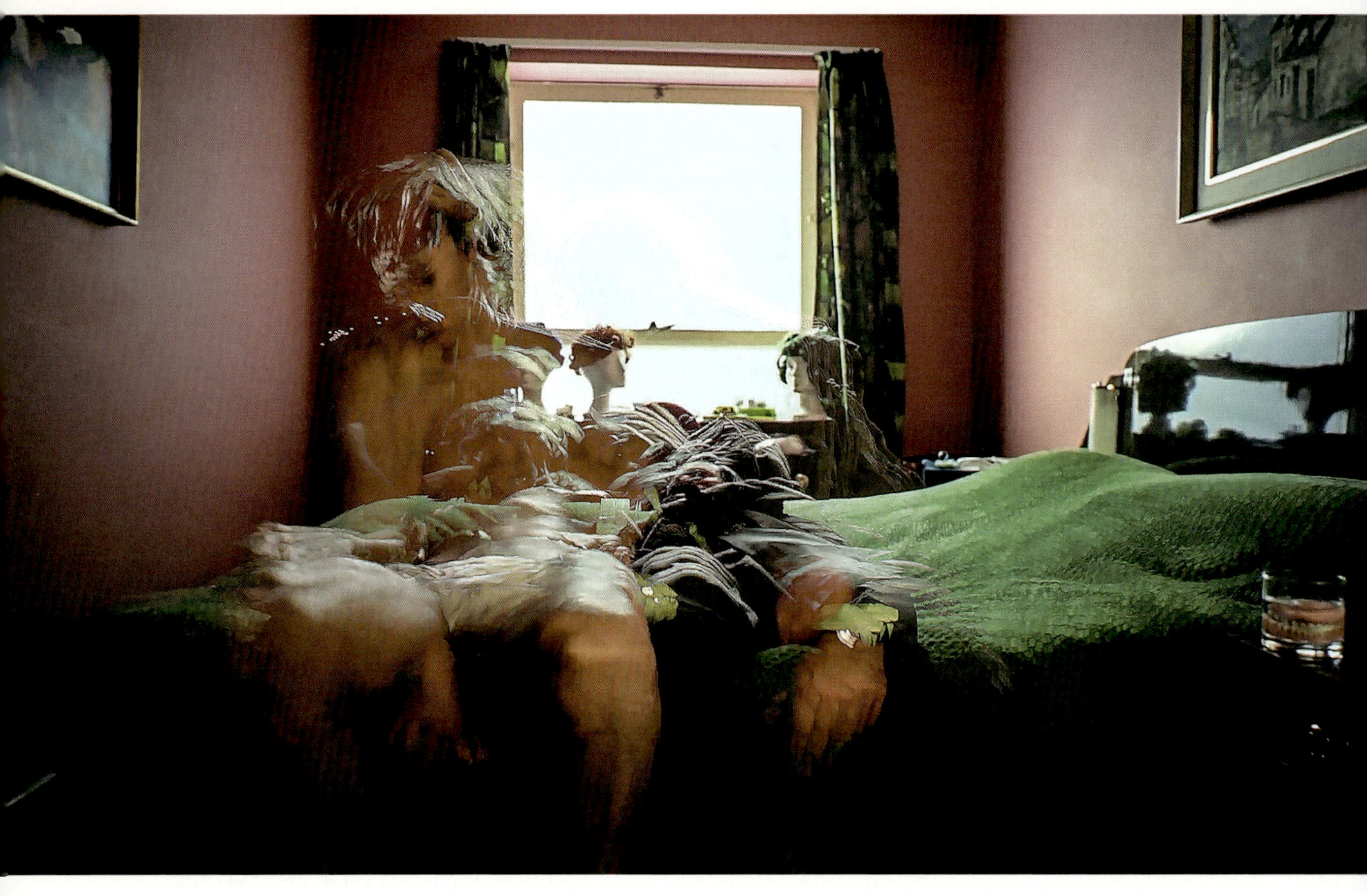

Just a Hard Rain #17,
2014. Digital drawing.

Agamben turns to Martin Heidegger: towering twentieth-century philosopher. Controversial in every way. Influential in every way. Sure, I read some Heidegger, difficult, but enjoyed his words more.

Being, Being-in-the-world, truth can be won, concealing and unconcealing, Time, being-towards-DEATH.

But really Heidegger simply opened me to have conversations with aAron, secret hero of all of this: friend. Healer or mystic doesn't do him justice. No words available yet, but, soon, we will simply say visionary or bodhisattva. Heidegger orients me to think about Being, but aAron reoriented my Being. Thank you, friend.

aAron, our conversations over the past year are written in all of these pages.

Heidegger says

// the stone is wordless; the animal is poor in world; and man is world-forming //

He says, the animal is caught in its perceptions, only behaving, and never in a world, yet it is out in the open: the flow of becoming, moment to moment. The human is world-generating with the inward turn of Self-awareness, Self-storying. This Self lays like a trap and never lets the human step into the pure space of the open. The human is a closed loop, split into many parts,

a gradient of Being

and the animal is one >> | << in the open—a being before Being, entering into the flow of becoming, moment to moment, breath to breath.

For the human, the creation of the Self is to have something to dissolve, for the narratological arc of becoming, to *become-animal, to have somewhere to step from into the open: journey. Expanding out of our worlding chrysalis, feeling the warm air, the sheltering magnetic field, finding our place in it all*

—consciousness, life, cosmos, eternity, infinity, connection.

Being

For us, the journey into the open is to develop practices, find a Charon that ferries you past these traps: Self, storying, ego, Default-Mode Network. All the illusions that mediate Being. The convincing hallucination. One dissolves the waking hallucination and enters into the pure space of Being,

Becoming,

the open.

But one does not step out into the open. One must go on a journey that is there for every human. Paths are cut but one must find their own trail into the abyss.

This journey only goes down, through your feet, through the ground, through the molten core of iron at the centre of the Earth, out into space,

through the moon, the sun,

the supermassive black hole at the centre of our galaxy,

and into the hinterlands of the mind.

There you will gaze into the abyss and make a gesture at it: art, a sensation, an opening. And with enough luck, the abyss will gaze into you and return a gesture. Send a sensation up your spine, making your hair stand on end, expanding the infinite space of consciousness a little further, or it might show you primordial images of your ancestral heritage,

awe.

You sense these sensations in your mind and body, this exchange otherwise, in a way that bypasses linearity, mortality, coherence, reason, language, and restructures your world-generating capacity, reorienting your Being, concealing or unconcealing. A cycle of birth, death, and rebirth, moment to moment, being to being across the cosmic expanse of Being and Time.

The journey into the open is a healing journey. It is an authentic spiritual journey. Waking up from the dream. Then falling into the bath of actualization: of lucid dreaming.

Our origin is the source of our essence. To be born is spontaneous. Life is a spontaneously unfolding expression to come to Know itself. You begin to Know through strife that provokes you out into the open. Presenting the always waiting abyss in spontaneous death in strife with spontaneous life. Learning how to die through abyssal confrontation, provoking you to learn how to live, Be, flow: becoming. To become is to be spontaneously reborn—origin.

Alignment.

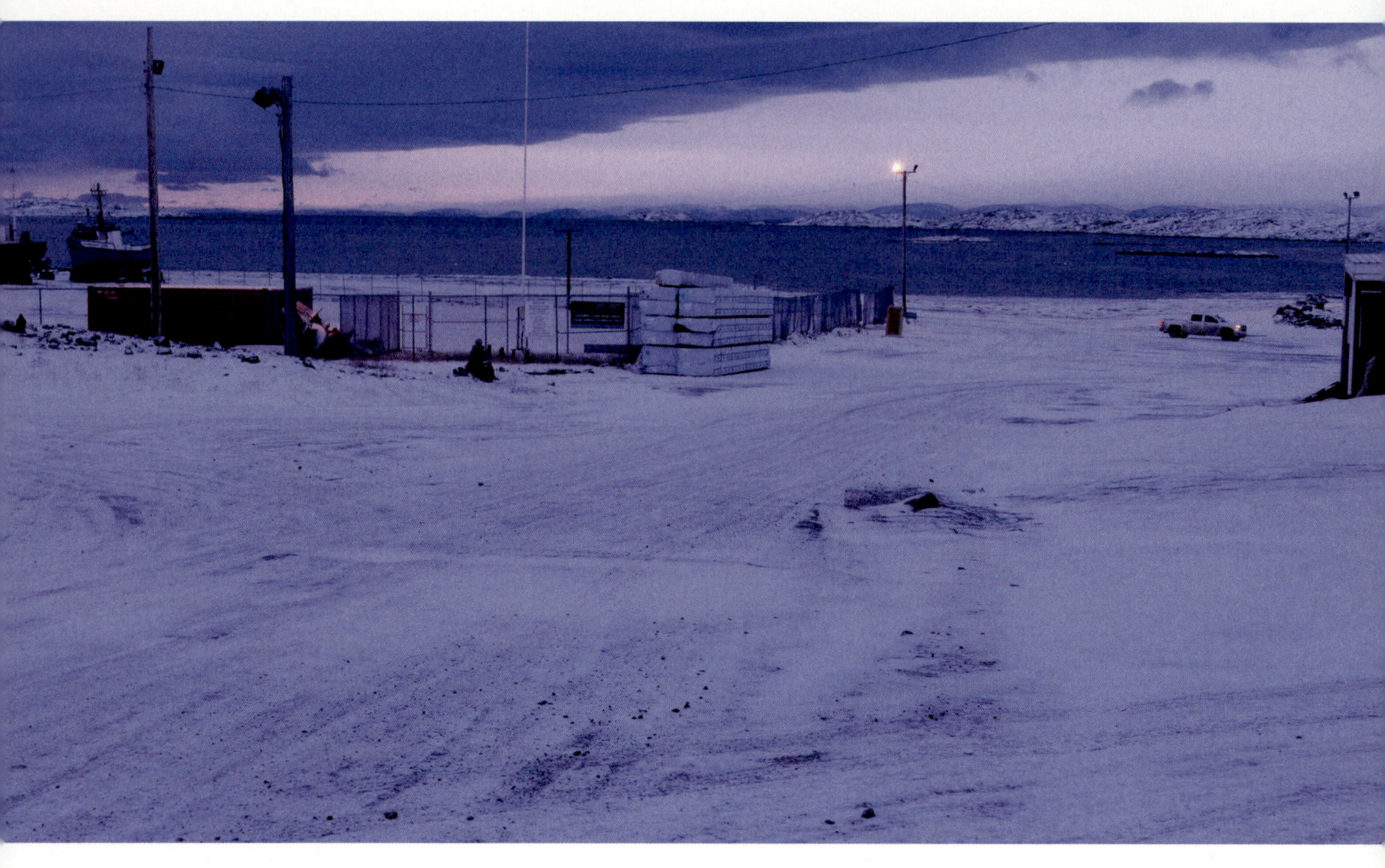

Morning light in Iqaluit,
Nunavut, October 2016.

I wake up. A fog of mood stabilizers, antipsychotics, anxiety pills, and sleeping meds presses on me, concealing Being. Even with all these sedatives I can't roll back to sleep. What am I doing here again?

I get up, put on my winter gear. Gloves and a hat this time as well. I grab my camera and walk outside. The peeking sun was casting a light of deep blues and purples, painting everything. I walk down the impassable path, to the bay.

NO TRESPASSING.

I take some photos, breathe in the morning air, unconcealing, even for a moment. Feeling a different sensation. Something within,

down
and down.
The feeling of feelings. The feeling
that something is about to happen.
A rod in Walter De Maria's *Lightning*
Field. Potential. I don't yet understand
this sensation. It courses through
me, guiding my hand as I look
and shoot.

No need for a cab. The high school is within walking distance. And so I walk and take photos on the way. I climb up a hill and walk through untouched snow to the edge of a small bluff. I see the city and out to the airport. I see the lunar landscape rolling and rolling. The air has finally woke me up.

I go into the high school and knock the snow off my boots. It's warm inside. Hard to imagine anything could be warm when the air cuts the way it does. What powers this heat?

I see Jennifer, my new friend. She asks me to go to a session with her and we sit together.

I haven't been in a high school classroom in fourteen years. The desks still fit. The walls are covered in formulas and posters. It feels like any other classroom. I haven't had this sensation in so long.

The speaker gets up.

Photovoice: we will go around and visually reflect on the school and the lingering theme of suicide. Then we will come back and narrate it to see the collective themes that emerge.

This is my workshop. The workshop I had planned, the one I was going to stumble through. I know I can't do it now.

She is a good presenter, and I'm interested in seeing what my photovoice session would have been like, so Jennifer and I go around the school to reflect and make images.

I look through round submarine windows. The contrast between the white snow outside and the grey walls inside is beyond my eye's apprehension.

I walk down the halls and see art everywhere. I see images of trauma, and messages of hope and healing.

I see art, quilting, and beading rooms.

I stand there engaged with a quilt hanging on a wall. Messages from students that had survived a loved one's suicide. All sewn into the quilt.

One message reads

Mom...I miss you so much. Thanks for the years you were able to share with me.

I slip

Elliot

baby Mary

I am so sorry

I slip

down

MORNING LIGHT, PAINTING PURPLE

breathe in

breathe out

NO TRESPASSING

I'll watch my step.

My feet are lead. My heart is lead. All directions are down.

Wisdom. When to use knowledge and when not to. This child, their wisdom.

MOM, MISS
THANKS
YEARS, SHARE

I can read the signs

Holy Mary, golden Ellie

I don't understand it yet but that message is reorienting my Being. Unconcealing. Even if just for a moment.

A sound wavering in perception. An ancient sound. A sound from some shared space. The depths of Being from the depths of a soul incarnate.

up

My mind pulls up and up and

I turn around and see a small amphitheatre: a stage surrounded by comfortable couches. Students assembling. Kids with instruments. Two girls facing each other, maybe less than a foot apart: throat singing.

Wow.

Power. Each breath and sound pushes air and power into the other's breath and sound. Back and forth.

breathe in   breathe out

meditation

present   merging   a column of air that is one with its breath

The kind of breathing and Being that makes your hair stand on end. The prickling sensation that wakes you up from a dream.

BOOM

I turn my head to the right slightly. Two students a few feet from each other. Looking into each other, past their eyes, into a space I don't yet understand. They begin to fuse as they beat their drums and dance. The throat singing continues and BOOM BOOM BOOM.

I slip

I slip

I slip

//

Holy! Holy! Holy! Holy! Holy! Holy! Holy! Holy! Holy! Holy! Holy! Holy!

The World is holy! The soul is holy! The skin is holy!

Everything is holy! Everybody's holy! Everywhere is holy! Everyday is in eternity! Every person is an angel!

Holy Frobisher Bay holy Edmonton holy CAMH holy Canada holy the VISIONS

holy the hallucinations holy the miracles holy the mind holy the abyss!

Holy Ellie   holy Candace   holy Mary Mom Dad!

Holy forgiveness! Mercy! Charity! Faith! Holy! Ours! Bodies! Suffering! BEING!

Holy the supernatural extra brilliant intelligent kindness of the open!

//

Holy children of Iqaluit.

Holy child's mom.

Jennifer stands beside me.

did you get any good photos?

Holy incarnation.

We go back into the classroom and sit down, like children.

We start narrating our images and Jennifer volunteers to write them down. She has nice writing.

I gaze out the rounded windows, slipping into a daydream, connections beyond the land.

Where were we, mom?
hospital my grave
her, child death
so much hunger tubes spilling everywhere
together
The comfort of a mother

We speak of Charon.

✳madness✳visions✳psychedelics✳meditation✳

Many of us are looking, but can't find the ferry—yet.

We don't live or die, but float, to paraphrase Dylan.

Or: we live and die, and so swim, surf, and breathe the waking dream.

Of course, one Charon is waiting for all of us, every single one. It has woven itself throughout this book, woven itself into Being, into my Being, into all our Beings. You know it as well as I do, you feel it, too, that gravity well pulling on you, the infinite black hole, that bottomless pit where all directions are d

o

w

n

DEATH

Quick, cover your eyes, don't look back! Not that death needs light or radiation or electromagnetism to warp our spirits, to pull on Being. I am watching this unfold in Elliot, this black hole of death. She senses it. She doesn't know it, yet, but she is coming to Know it in herself, moment to moment, breath to breath, as she grows with death. It is pulling on her, insisting that there is more to this, there is something outside of this, something beyond this.

To look, sense, dissolve, awaken.

Whatever that means, to a six-year-old.

This engagement with the abyss is hanging in every room—and when we acknowledge it, when we open ourselves to death's presence, we are more alive than ever. On the edge of a mountain, falling out of a plane, leaving psilocybin to kill that thing you call yourSelf; death as a gamma-ray burst from another galaxy. Incineration, evaporation, sublimation: mass converts to energy and rides the sacred light beam.

We have phenomenological accounts from this abyss—madness, psychedelics, visions, meditation—and so we know that it isn't only nothing but also everything.

To enter the purest space, the openest of the open, you cross that final river and, simply, clearly, easily, die.

Die now or die later.

Death is patient. This ferryman is in no rush. But bring a coin or you're in for a stormy ride. The coin you need is here, in life, we set sail, it's just over here, out here, in the open, it's waiting for you—to dissolve.

Don't worry, there'll be no more of that. No body or mind, bliss or suffering, life or death, just,

One.

Being.

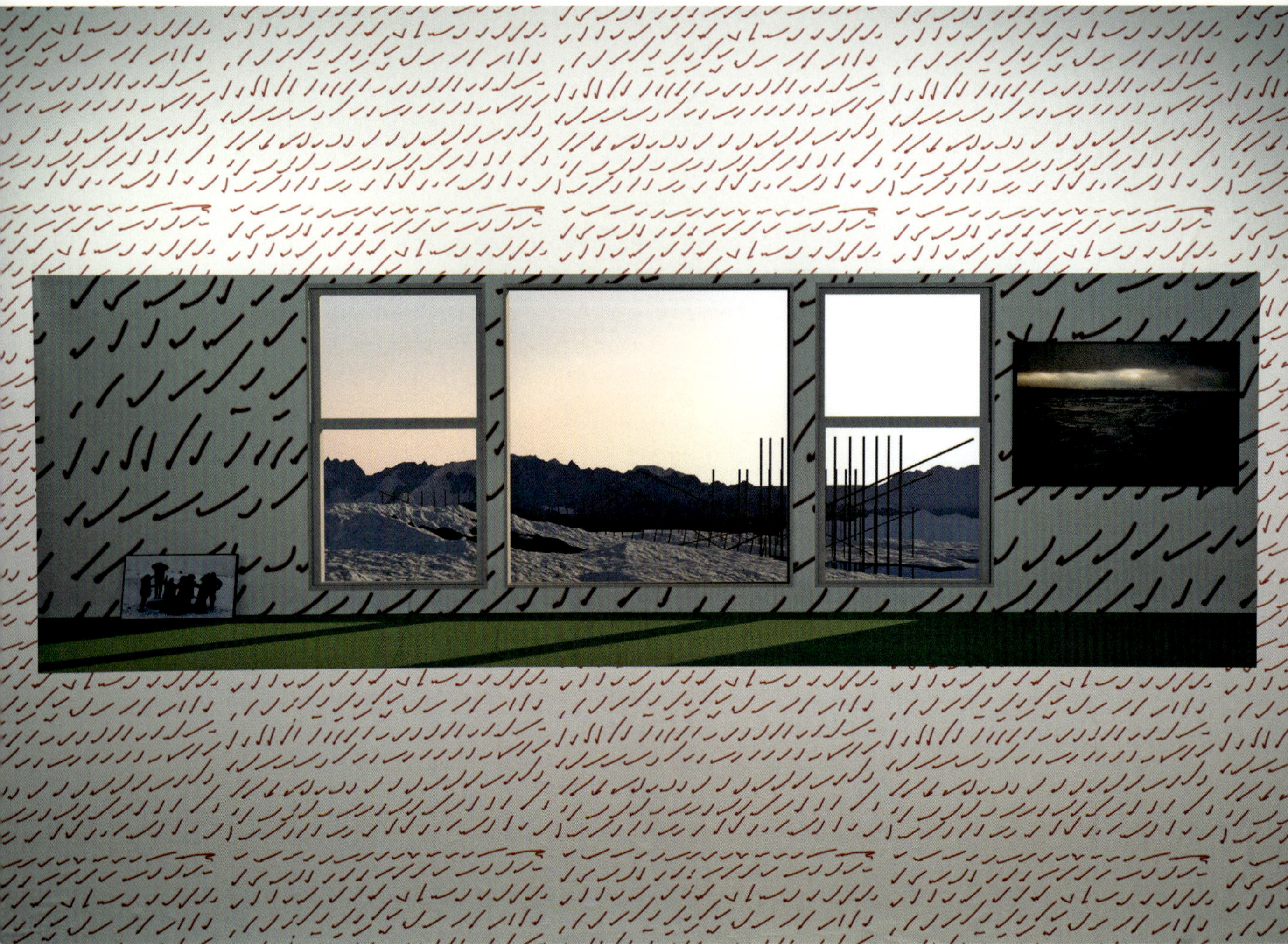

Dwelling Otherwise, 2018. Photographic installation, 14' × 14'.

A DRY CITY

It was cold in Iqaluit, something a Canadian should be used to but it made the ground harder than hard. I flowed in and out of conference sessions, never finding a footing. The night before was a celebration of art: Inuit fashion and music. Beings expressing themselves, falling, and opening. I bear witness and feel something I don't understand yet. Art, spirituality, and Being, one. These kids have power. Marks in the air.

I walk around the city, taking pictures, sensing sensations.

It was too cold to walk home so I called a cab

I say:

where is the nearest liquor store?

Driver:

dry city. No alcohol for years. Too much damage. Too much loss. There are ways to get a bottle of vodka for two hundred dollars.

He says you could buy a beer if you order a meal at a restaurant.

Thiry-two years of comfort in a small suburb in Alberta.

I look at the driver. Harder than hard

—loss, addictions, suicides—

all bursting everywhen, collapsing in my synaptic cleft,
radiating sensations of the gravity well pulling on my Being.
Too many sensations. I need to dissolve. Some solvents to
block up that cleft.

He says

this isn't the way his people wanted to live, this isn't the way they are supposed to live. But the presence of the Canadian government and the pressing force of the South is everywhere. It's not doing anyone any good.

Later, I leave my hotel.

I turn left at Federal Road and Niaqunngusiariaq. Walking into a mist to become a mist.

Table for one.

I sit in the restaurant, order a meal, and order a beer. I guess this is why everyone had bottles of vodka in their bags. I should have done some research. Sixty dollar pasta and twenty dollar beer. But everything comes from somewhere else.

I sit with myself and listen to the room. I hear two men talking about hunting and how the ice is changing. Lost trails. Distinctions where there were no distinctions before.

They eat fish and are

Holy.

I see people sitting with multiple meals in front of them so they can continue to order beers.

Holy.

I see married couples enjoying meals together.

Holy.

I see people on dates.

Holy.

I feel the presence of love as life and death hang in the room with us in this land beyond the land.

A voice once unclear:

Canada.

// When will you be angelic?
When will you take off your clothes?
When will you look at yourself through the grave?
//

Sun and Moon, 2020.
11-minute film created
with Jonathan Kawchuk.

In January 2020, I read Heidegger's *The Origin of the Work of Art* and it says:

// Art creates space for spaciousness //

Then early June, two nights ago, aAron and Jonathan Kawchuk, musician and friend, come over to my backyard: social distance. Jonathan and I had just completed *Sun and Moon* and we're screening it together for the first time on two TVs side by side. We pass the keyboard and mouse back and forth to get it running, sanitizing our hands after each pass. We wait till the sun sets at 9:56 p.m. so all we see is *Sun and Moon*. And we do.

After watching it we sit back and stare up into the black, clouded over sky, swatting the mass of mosquitoes looking for life. Before, while waiting for less light, we watch episode five of *Midnight Gospel*. In the prison of our repeating mistakes and dis-orientations, they talk about Indra's Net, a field of consciousness where the impression of an individual comes at sites of overlapping connections, nodes, that reflect *everything*, the entirety of everything is held in each node—*radiant jewel*.

And so we talk about consciousness and stories, old tired stories that aren't usable to think with anymore.

We talk about America. We talk about the stories George Floyd lived, and the stories that led a man to kneel on a being's neck and squeeze the life out of him.

We talk about revelation and meditation and psychedelics.

Art does create space for spaciousness. On this night I feel an expanse of connection. The infinite netting of the universe, three nodes of connection beside each other on the prairies of Alberta, *reflecting Being, reflecting each other, reflecting the whole of the cosmos*

and all of everything.

Watching an interview with Carl Jung, vision-seeker that SEES visions, they ask,

// Do you believe in God? //

And Jung said, // I do not believe, I Know. //

It hit me like a tsunami, to Know, not think, or believe, or hope, but Know. I have many degrees, learning a lot, maybe know a bit too. But that intellectual knowing happens in the prefrontal cortex that gets stored in the temporal, occipital, and parietal cortices. These are the most evolutionarily recent additions to the organ of the brain, in their size and density, unique to humans. They allow all the higher-level processing that helps us think, ruminate, plan, and execute all the things that become bank accounts, missiles, and carbon. Where our ego or Default-Mode Network mediates our Being,

concealing and concealing,

constricting this hallucination, so does all this explicit knowing. It adds another hallucination to the perceptual hallucination we can't seem to awaken from, a hallucination that is always there. That we can't even remember we are in anymore.

The kind of Knowing Jung speaks of comes from the abyss, the strife between suffering and love experienced before Being: Burkean sublime, awe, ecstasy, revelation. This is nonrational, nonlinear, nonlinguistic, noncoherent Knowing, bypassing all those parts of the brain that make us human. In a sense, you *become-animal*, shedding the Self, our humanness, entering into the open, *a being with and within Being.* The reorientation that happens during this is Knowing. The reorientation is teaching, restructuring how you world, which then tells you stories otherwise that change your waking hallucination. Aware of the dream, mindfulness, expressing and taking pleasure in the lucid opportunities of incarnation. There is no thinking with this teaching, reasoning it out, but, instead, the confidence to simply

KNOW.

The visionary artist is a way to Knowing, a thin place, between this realm and the next, finding Charons, crossing and falling into the depths, dissolving and merging, emerging, screaming for breath, in the open. No longer human but simply returning to the ancient form of a being, now before and within Being. Free of all the boundaries and distinctions that aren't really there, layers on the hallucination. Entering into the pure space, blistered, no one. Sensing all the strife between human and animal/being, suffering and joy, conscious and unconscious, body and mind, waking hallucinations and Being, concealment and unconcealment, knowing and Knowing, and all can be won through sensing this strife, being with it.

Only in the pure space of the open can we come to Know. To Know incarnation, merging and healing the strains and stresses of being in a body, with a mind, in a field of consciousness, the Being of Being.

Last day of the conference: Saturday, October 29, 2016.

My workshop: 1 p.m. Following the keynote.

My flight: 4 p.m. Back to Ottawa, the Canada I know
knew.

That dinner with holy people moves me. The singing and dancing children move me. It summons sensations I have no names for. Exploding, collapsing under its weight, held in suspense, disbelief, and love. I get back to my hotel room and slip

notebook, writing

arts-based research

Diane Conrad, Professor, University of Alberta, illuminator

We are fundamentally creative and aesthetic beings.

Other ways to Knowing: art, expression, the abyss

pause, some shared language. Right. Qualitative research.

raise consciousness
identifying areas that need work
give voice to those without a voice
promote dialogue
evoke multiple meanings

Arts-based research becomes a method to enrich an ongoing conversation by making visible, intensifying sensation, and engaging social change.

No matter our training, no matter our creativity, we all can contribute.

Image theatre

Thank you, David Diamond.

We are all here thinking about suicide. Our theme will be

visualizing a way through

We will make living sculptures, one gesture to the abyss after another, then

maybe the abyss will make a gesture back, send a sensation up our spine, illuminating, provoking, comforting, terrifying, loving. Some collective idea will emerge,

a way through.

We are here to fell a clearing, create a World, a free region to inhabit, a place to be vulnerable, filled with connection, inclusive enough to gaze into the abyss, and, with enough luck, the abyss will gaze back into us. Maybe we can tell some stories otherwise from this exchange.

12:30. I get into the classroom and sit at the teacher's desk. Looking at the walls: formulas, life cycles of spontaneously unfolding beings. Desks in rows all pointing in one direction, forward. Power.

I take out chairs and push the tables back, creating a circle.

We are part of a larger conversation.

I write on the whiteboard

Brad Necyk

bnecyk@ualberta.ca

Writing Suicide

Then, new title

Visualizing a way through

I sit at the teacher's desk and look at my notebook. I practice under my breath.

POWER OUTAGE. Backup generators, flickering lights.

1 p.m.: no one is here.

1:10 p.m.: still no one.

Jennifer flies into the room

where is everyone?

Relief

I don't know

No one at either of our sessions.

Maybe a cosmic intervention. I have no idea what I am doing.

1:30 p.m.: loud steps, lots, coming down the hall.

Fifteen people, or so, fill the room. They say the keynote was delayed because of the power outage.

We sit in a circle. I introduce myself and what I have felt over the past few days. I tell them about arts-based research, image theatre, and how I hope we can try, even if just a glimpse, to visualize a way through. I don't know it yet: the pure space of the open.

I measure my moves against David's, but slowly I slip, less measuring, more spontaneity.

We get started.

Half of the room steps back behind the tables. They will be our witnesses. Worlding us in place. Others sit at the edge of their seat. Holy everyone.

will someone go up and make a shape with their body?

A gesture to the abyss.

Gesture

can someone else make a shape in response?

Hello abyss. Can you see us?

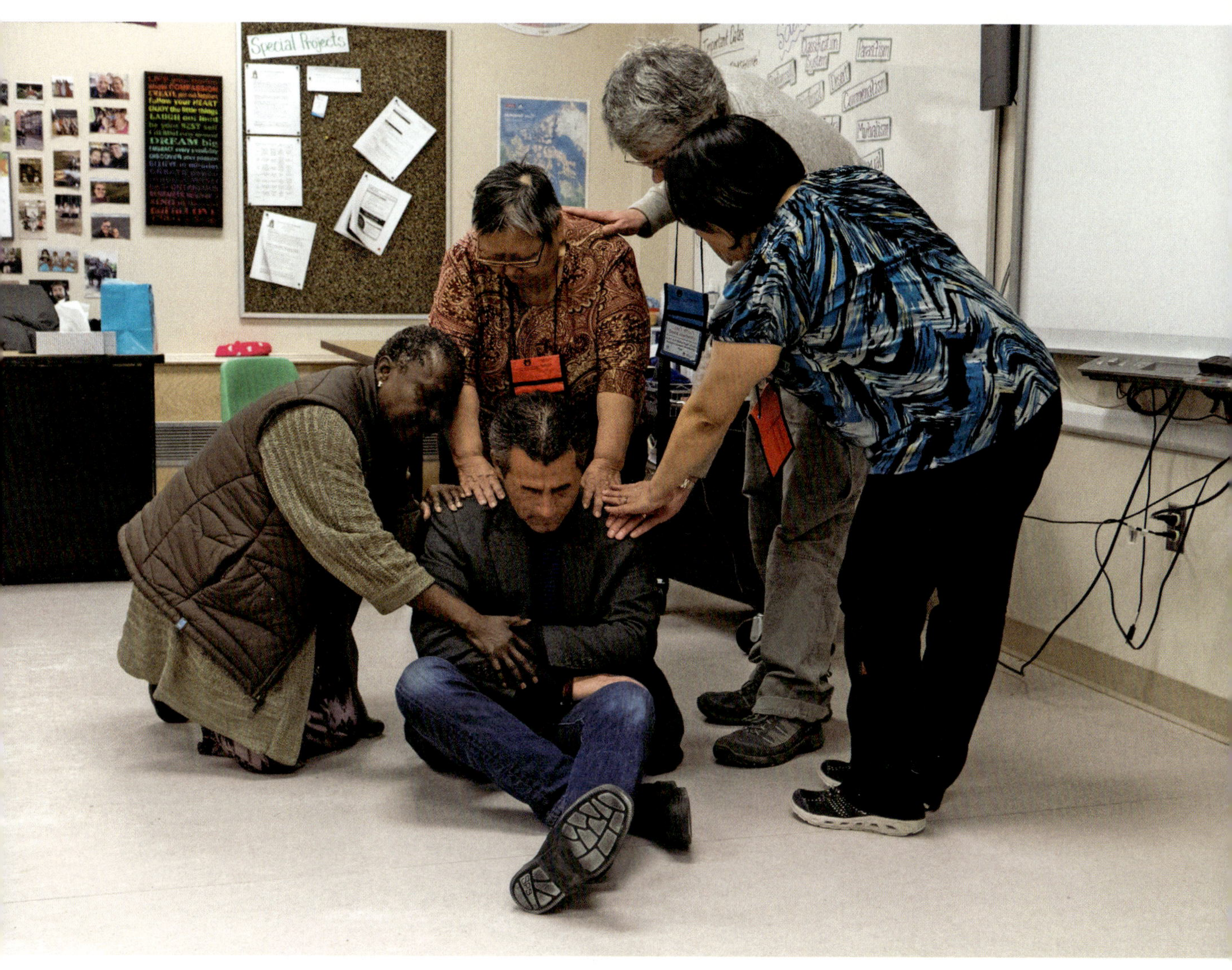

Living sculpture from Visualizing a Way Through workshop, Iqaluit, October 2016.

—ancient sensation

Okay. Let's exchange.

Five bodies.

Five nodes in a school, the lightning rod of potential.

We pause and I take a picture.

Spontaneous image. *Because life is a spontaneous unfolding, and this conference is celebrating life.*

can anyone narrate this image?

we are in it together.

Sensation makes my hair stand on end. A subjective truth that has objective reality because someone has realized it. *We* realize it.

We make a second image. Photo.

Stay spontaneous. David enters my mind:

> does anyone have an image in their minds? Can you get up and sculpt it with the people in this room?

Mouth moves:

> does anyone have an image in their minds? Can you get up and sculpt it with the people in this room?

Thanks, David.

A woman does. Person after person, story after story, gesture after gesture. Unfolding.

Hello abyss. Here we are. Bare.

Abyss, now when will you take off your clothes? When will you look at yourself through the grave?

Holy! Holy! Holy!

I look at the clock. Only fifteen minutes left. I ask if they would like to come outside, to create these images in the landscape so present in everything we are hoping for. They agree. We bundle up and head out the back door.

THICK SNOW, OCCLUDING EVERYTHING.

Maybe this is just right. We look on my camera at each image and recreate them. We are laughing and stumbling to navigate the landscape and the snow. Life and death hang in the corner, but we are now a spontaneous unfolding, not Brad and the next person and the next, but one. We move and breathe together. Hot breath misting out our mouths, warming the air.

in and out.

(Top) *Together*, 2016.
(Middle) *Hope*, 2016.
(Bottom) *Are You Listening?*, 2016.

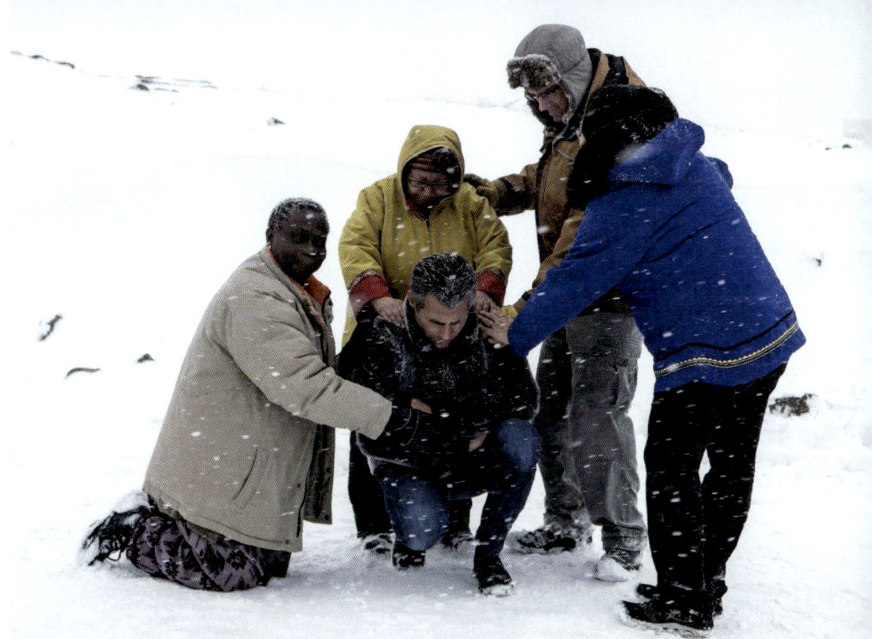

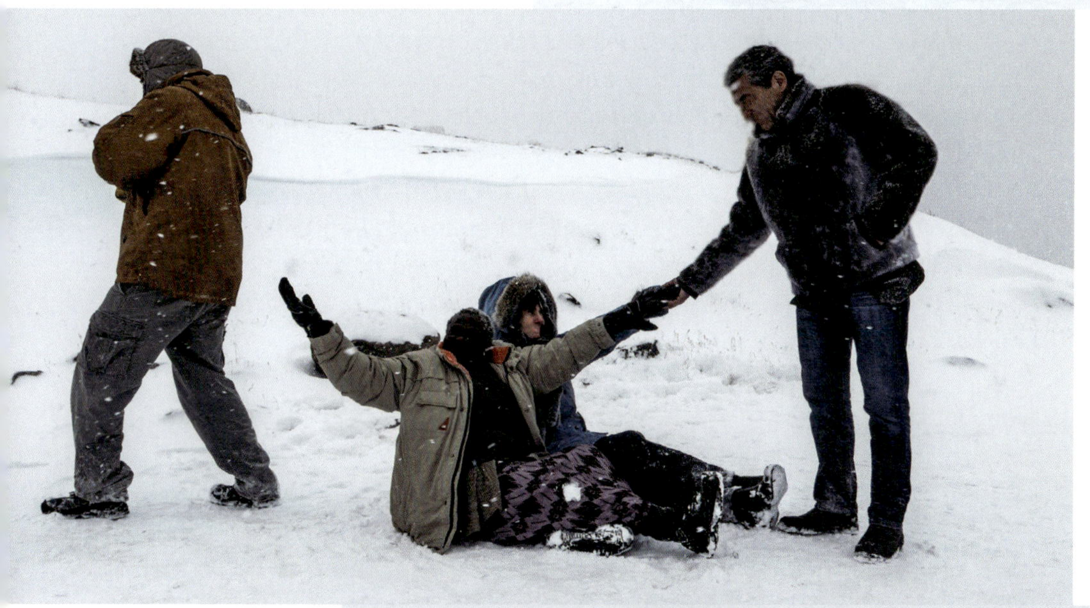

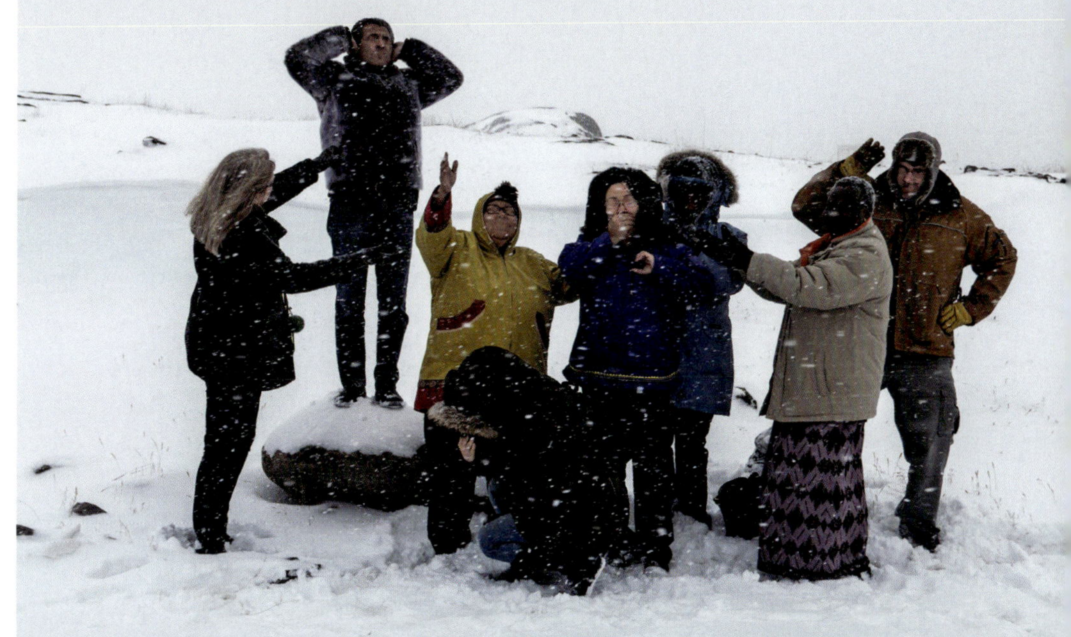

Hope is holy. These children are holy. This land beyond the land is holy. Sensation arises:

We share an experience, coarse and twisted, knotted, strung along a stretching expanse. It is a very ancient space we all inhabit, it's nested deep within each of us, deeper than genetic strands stretching across a geological timescale of billions of years, one that is in a space for communal kinship. We are all in it together.

We finish and I never see any of them again. I feel that we have done something special. *That life is spontaneous, that we are spontaneous, that we allowed the universe to unfold in that moment:*

KNOWING.

I feel a sense of something I am not ready to understand. It is a kind of clarity, maybe a bit like love. I walk back to the hotel, collect my things, and head to the airport. The storm stops. The sky parts and our airplane lands with fresh people, ready to take in this town, these people, this land beyond the land.

Indra, your net is collecting mist in a land across time. I am gazing into a drop on it held in suspense: pulling from inside and pressing from outside. Balance. Perfection. I look closer. I see myself in the drop, I see all of Iqaluit in it. I am worlding it and it is worlding us. Collapsing each other's wave function to Be.

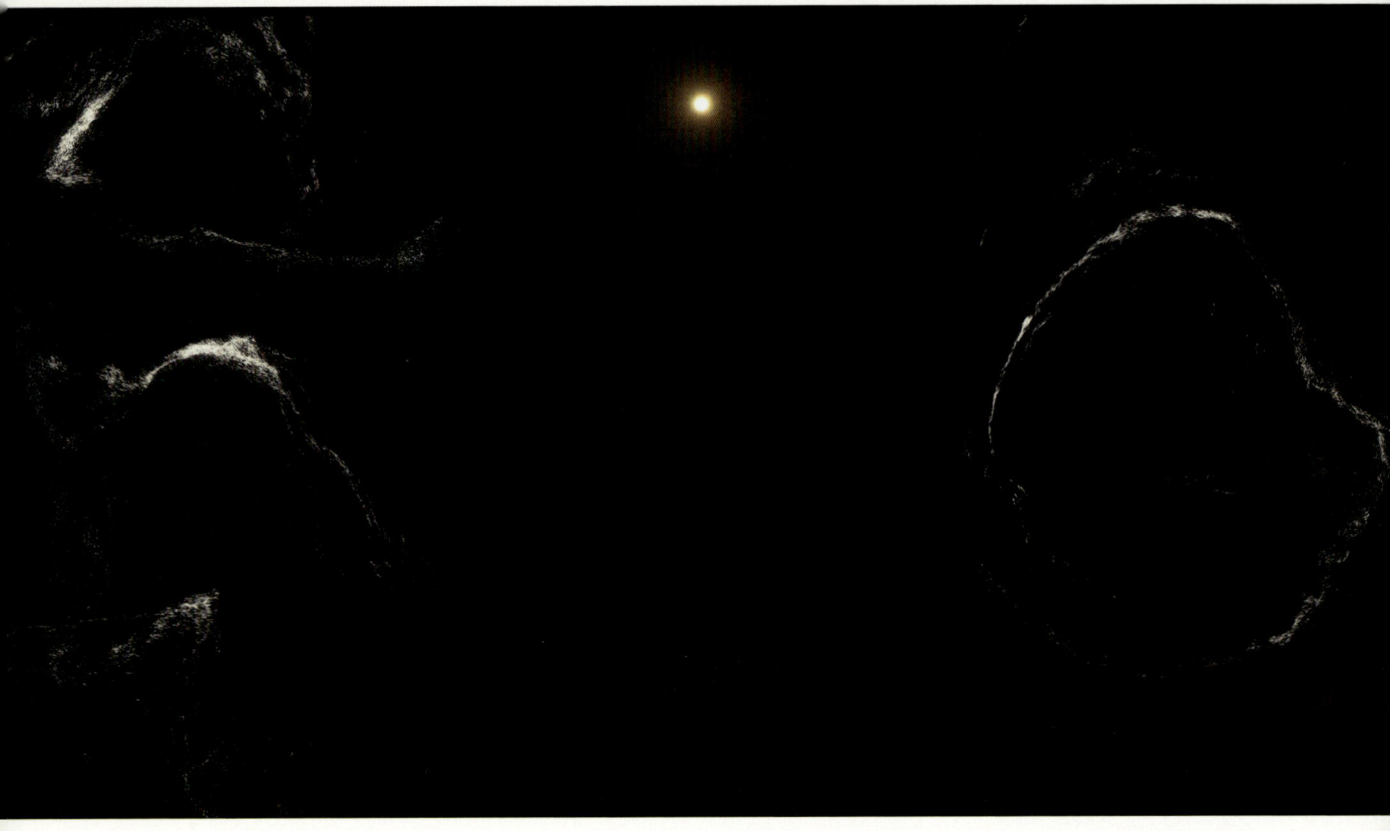

Kingdom of Illumination (the abyss), 2020–2021. 25-minute film created with Gary James Joynes.

The abyss is a state of consciousness, the plane you pass onto.
// Where the doors of perception have been cleansed and everything appears as it is, infinite //

The open ocean,
BEING ;;;

//

\\

You find a Charon.
\\ visions | madness | psychedelics | meditation //

breathe in breathe out

Then, caught in the raging ocean storm of life.
Caught in the rotation that pulls you down
and
down, >>
and so you fall into the whirlpool's event horizon, where nothing can return.

You might resist, of course you will resist. But soon there is nothing to be won, and so you fall, || *because falling is easier than resisting* ||

The blackness consumes and you live a million million lifetimes in the void, the thin place, the portal between worlds.
Bathing in the primordial sea.

After a cosmic epoch: light.
Something,
anything happens.

Faint:
collecting, exploding, rotating, blasting into infinity
and hoping for eternity.

In the darkness, you sense the sensations cresting at your feet. How long has that been here?

You continue to stare into the expanse,
the lone witness to the birth of a universe.

The ebb and flow continues at your feet as you gaze into the nothingness but cosmic ages of an infant universe.

<<stars supernovae white dwarfs neutron stars
black holes supermassive black holes galaxies quasars>>
the larger structure of the Greater Mind unfolding expressing
coming to Know itself you watch it all

There is nothing but waiting, nowhere to go, and so you continue to slip away, outside of time, outside of thoughts, outside of You. ~~You~~ have been here so long that the idea of You is like a dream.

And as ~~You~~ wake up you forget it,
like you do all your dreams.

Then, light. A sliver of light that gives birth to a horizon.
More light:
the dancing forms on the ocean that has been at your feet since the beginning of time.
~~You~~ see the stars that have collected across time, flickering.
Stars: pure becoming.
~~You~~ meditate on all of this as nobody.
The pure space.
The open.
And ~~You~~ see the full presentation of the universe, ~~You~~ see everything,
unconcealed,
glimpsing,

~~Your~~ mind flickers to Indra's Net.
Empty, emptied, emptiness.
Radiant jewel, mystical child
breathe in
breathe out
The most open openness
Allspace for spaciousness
Finding your place in it all.

ALIGNMENT
to the
ORIGIN

This is the beginning of how the abyss reorients ~~Your~~ Being.

, now an origin.

I

I sit.
I sat. I am sitting
again, now, New Year's Eve: 2020, 9:03 p.m.,
thinking about you,
I thought about you,
mom and dad.

Sitting in 2012 I write: to my left is a stack of photographs stamped on the back
July 1987
There are 76 with that stamp.
56 are from some day in July of an outdoor birthday party.
20 are from another birthday, my birthday, in a hospital kitchenette room.
The outdoor birthday is shared between my brother and I. We always share
one in the middle of our birthdays, less than two weeks apart: July. It's his first
birthday, will be my third.
I move away the day after his birthday this year.
Sunny, warm prairies lawn chairs, kids tables, swing set,
Blue, blue sky sandbox shed, brown short fence,
grass that tickles and itches a bit.
Kids, me, my brother are playing.
The dads, grandpa are drinking beer.
The moms, grandma are taking care of us.
then, there are a number of people I no longer know.
We eat hotdogs, drink milk, play, and open gifts.

My dad isn't in any of the photographs.

Some of the
pictures are from
his 6-foot height,
and, then some on
knee, some close
portraits. Of the
56 from that day
I am in 37. I wear a
green shirt with
yellow and blue
shorts hiked up
past my belly
button. This is
what my father

was looking at.
I am what my
father is looking at.
O Dad,
my dad,
I am looking
at you
now today,
Dad,
Parkinson's
then, stroke,
I am so sorry.
You are my
dad and
I love you.
You are who I am
looking at
I was who you were
looking at, that
summer July day.

In one photo you can see me laughing—
head up, back knees bent, butt sticking back.
In it,

you can see the outline of my colostomy bag that is trying to be hidden by my hiked shorts. It is surgically installed during Easter, and directly after this joint birthday party I am heading to the hospital to have it removed, along with parts of my intestines.

again, I look. I am what my dad is looking at. As I look at this photograph I am seeing what you were seeing. I think that is why there are so many photographs of me that day,

in case I died. I look at you Ellie, Mary. I am imagining looking through
my camera, at both of you, a different you
—knowing this might be over
, knowing that is what my dad is looking at,
as he hit the shutter up and down,
letting the light travelling 8 minutes
through the void of space,
1/30th of a second,
to transfer their heat, onto the burn of
the film.
And when I look at that photo, dad,
all I see is you, I see all of you,

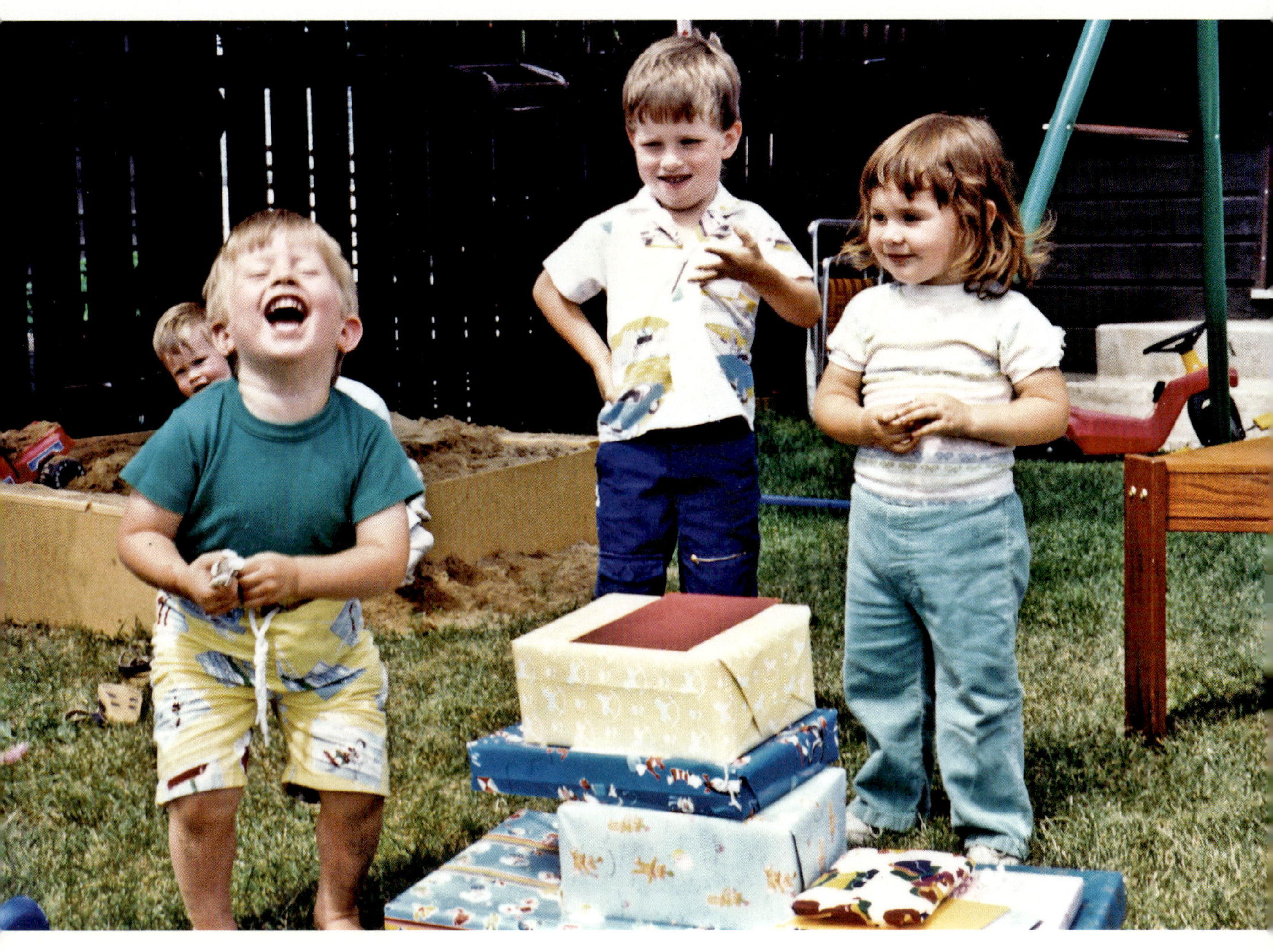

Me laughing.

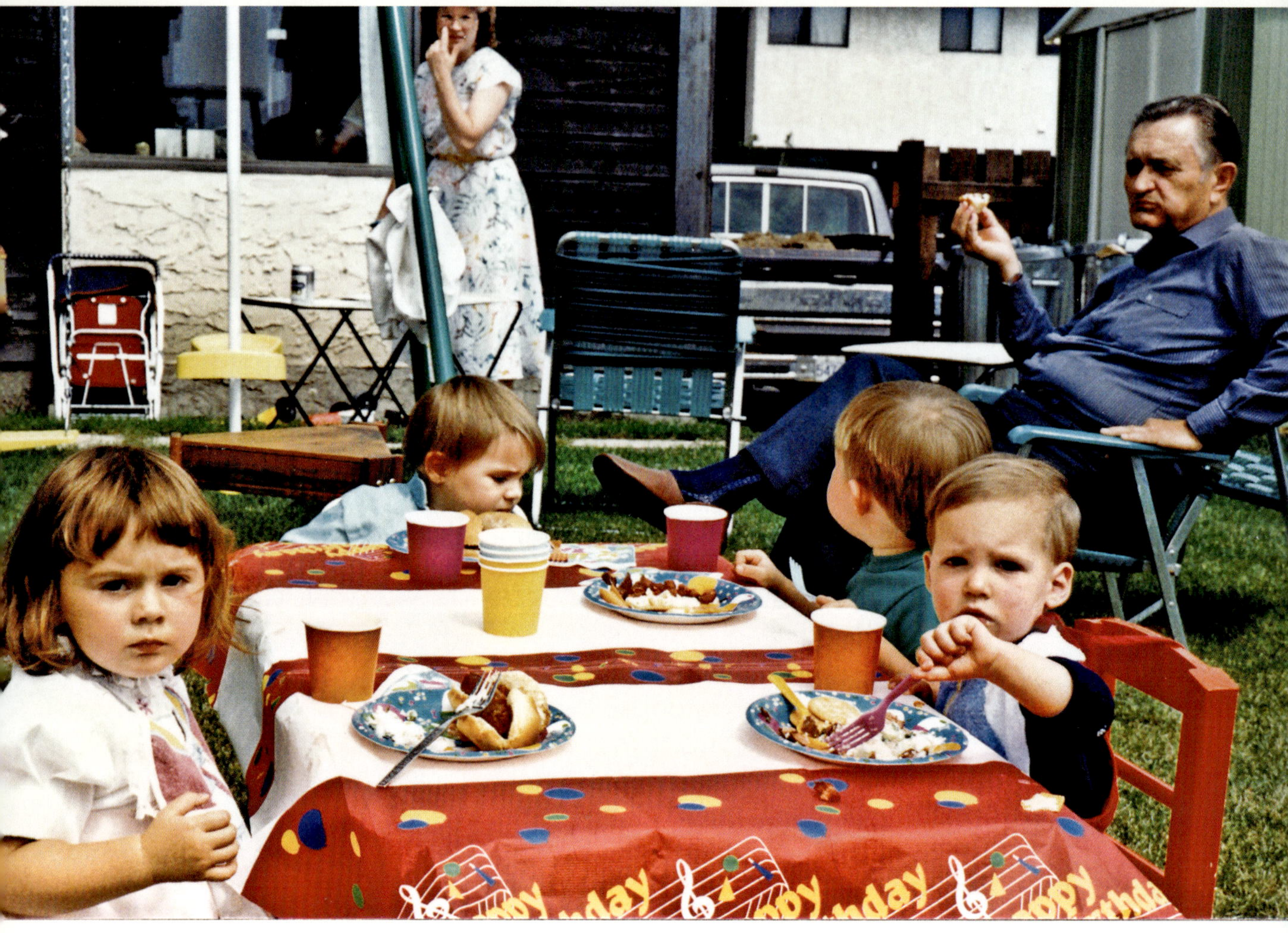

I am looking at you, Mom, from the kids' table.

a jewel on Indra's Net,
reflecting the whole of the cosmos
in yourself,
in this photo, looking at your child,
as I look at my child,
bringing in imaginary New Year's
at 8 p.m.,
now 10:34, everyone sleeping
as I am listening to the first Dylan song
you showed me: *Tangled Up in Blue*
when I was learning guitar at 20
and here I am, still dreaming of the sky
you and I always did feel the same
looking into distant stars
milky ways, late night comets
and I do with Ellie Mary,
always with you,
hammering and hammering visions,
strumming and strumming choruses.
I look at this photo and see me,
I look at this photo and see you,
I look at this photo and see us,
reflecting each other,
reflecting all of everything,
everything is held in ~~you~~, in ~~me~~,
O Dad, I will miss you, I will miss
looking at you.

Then there's this one photograph of me where there are
three kids looking around at the kids' table,
my grandfather in the mid-ground staring at me while chewing,
and my mom in the background looking at me while rubbing her eye.
I am looking at you, Mom.
You are looking at me, Mom.

A flash of heat, travelling 8 minutes from the sun, reflecting off my mother's sad face and the back of my hair, entering the camera and burning onto the film capturing our gaze. That 1/30th of a second of heat as light is preserved on a Kodak print that is now reflecting and absorbing light from the fluorescent bulbs in my basement.

Splatting photons , of varying wavelengths, are bouncing around this room, most
missing my eye, but some are entering. Igniting my rods and cones, radiating in my synaptic clefts, dropping cascading

signals, vibrations, connections, connections,
reflections, taking all this heated noise, and world
this photograph,
my dad looking at me,
my mom looking at me,
now, me looking at us.

I don't remember this photograph,
my mom remembers though. I once ask her about this photograph and she imagines her footing at that party, at that moment, in that moment, before me, touching her eye, whether an itch, a compulsion or a tear, I don't know. She knows.

My head lays bare
she might remember my face
I look at you I remember your face
you remember our gaze
I remember our gaze. Earlier tonight, imaginary New Year's
you holding back tears
I am holding back tears as the sky folds over both of us
late winter night, not that far apart (when you think about it)
but forever apart COVID sometimes I look at you, on our calls,
my mom,
and I think back to this photograph, that exchange.
It is one of deep sadness to stand 15 feet from your child,
it is one of deep sadness to sit here, 1296 kilometres from you,
then,
with that light with those people there,
imagining soon the movement that will occur,
the movement occurring watching Dad, you get older
ending in that hospital,
in that room,
where I will lay bare,
where you will lay bare.
56 pictures in a few hours span. 37 of me.

II

The first photograph in the hospital is of me in a train conductor outfit wearing a birthday hat and standing in front of a door with a sign saying

Happy Birthday To You
and
I'm 3 Today
On my left hand is a hospital admittance bracelet.
I am smiling and have not yet had the surgery.

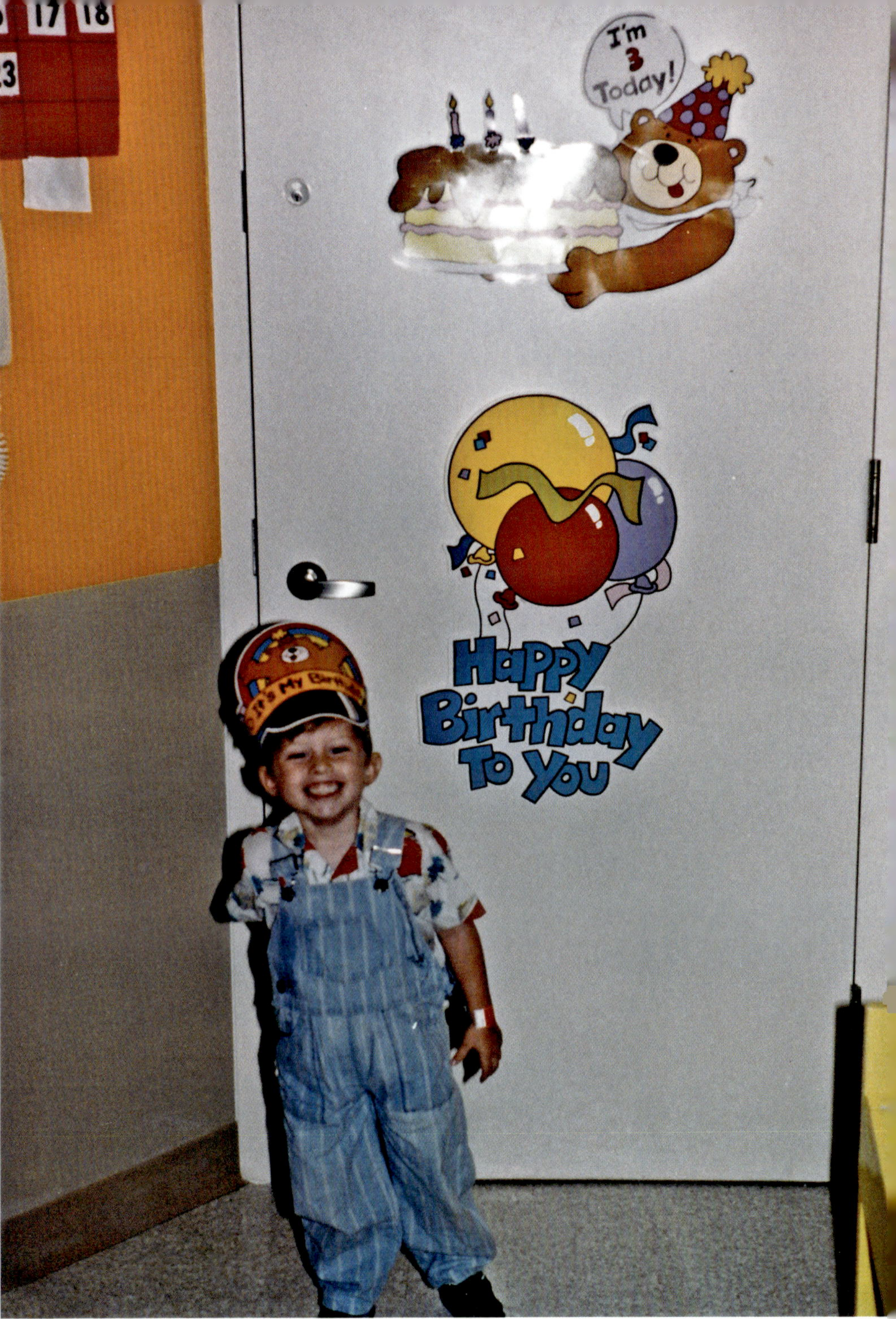

Happy birthday.

There is a group of half a dozen kids and their moms. My grandparents are there.

The room is a mix of a kitchenette and a playroom. There are toys and mats to sit on. There are tubes twisting everywhere, from kids noses,   from kids arms.

One girl has her foot caught around the tube of another kid, it wraps around his ears and into his nose.

There is another kid with an old IV cart that is big and blue, with a tube falling around the floor, wrapping around the room, wrapping around us, that runs into her hand, and this girl's hand is wrapped like an oven mitt, like my hands will be wrapped like an oven mitt, to not let us tear out the needles pressing pain pain pain in our arms. I never get used to needles being in my hands.

Another kid was in some strange stroller I have never seen since. He has a feeding tube attached to his nose and taped to the side of his face and he was sort of looking back at one of the adults, maybe his mom, looking for his mom.

Another kid has the same disease I do and is beginning the surgeries I started months before. He is in the photograph with his mom who is wearing a long-sleeve white shirt.

There is a picture of a doctor, maybe my doctor, and a nurse eating pieces of my cake.

All moms there, no dads, except my dad, omitted in photograph, but present as the photographer. These twenty fractions of a second recorded are identical impressions of my dad's visual experience, at that moment,   in that moment, I am in that moment, then and now. It is with his left eye closed as he uses his right eye to look in the viewfinder, to move, to look, to shoot. There are no photographs by him on his knee or any close portraits, just distanced, fully standing shots.

A distance felt throughout the room, then, now in this photograph.

O Dad, when I first write this story in 2012, I was not yet a father. When I look at these photos and write then I see it one way. Now as a father, sitting here on New Year's Day, outside, grey sky, cool fingers typing, looking through the glass at my daughters playing, I see it a different way

again, I look over a chasm, imagining the abyss, emotions summoning the abyss,
I look back across the abyss at my girls,

I don't remember this party   I don't remember the surgery,
hollow memories
I do sense the pressure of a ten-foot needle in my arm
the pressure of the gas mask the nurses are pressing on my face
the pressure of the air is different

the smell is chemical   there is no oxygen   each breath feels like
breathing in an ocean
flooding my lungs   dizzy dizzy dizzy   falling into the void of nothing
the empty space of anesthesia   the space where you no
longer exist
empty   emptied   emptiness
scrambling sensations of terror,   O Mom, where is my mom?
they take off the mask because I am screaming   Mom
they put it back on and I scream
they talk to themselves that they will have to give me a needle
I scream
the doctor looks at the whites of my eye and says it will be over soon
they put on the mask and I cry in resignation

I don't remember waking up   but I can create an image
based on all the other surgeries I can remember   I can feel
they cut me from one side of my pelvis to the next   I lift my orange
winter puffer coat
then shirt
and look at this scar   now,   pale yellow/orange tear and memory
they took out the dead part of my colon and the plastic from the colostomy
weave and knot my intestines back together
unsure if they would grow back together
that might be how I would die
then use six metal staples to close me
but not close me completely
I would be left partially open
to not trap infection
I cannot eat for
ten days
as my body tries
to repair
as my body tries
to heal
as I still try to heal
writing these words
imagining,
summoning
these terrible
memories
these terrible
sensations

this unimaginable fate
that has me, over
and over
remembering and
remembering
following these
thoughts
these sensations
that brings me to
the abyss
before the abyss
to lay with life
and death
    hung in the room
my body fighting the
pull of
    entropy
then experiencing
the miracle
    of life, healing
weaving and
knotting
    my intestines
    with
    my bipolar,
    crashing
    my memories,
    now
    connecting
    myself
    to myself, then
    to remember
    suffering
    to be with
    suffering
    to be suffering
    to see suffering is
        universal
    awakening
    compassion
    awakening love
    for you, me

for each hollow
apparition
        I scream at
        beat me
        hands at
but I think of
your smile
        , Mom
the positive love
you
        send to
        everyone
and I think of you,
Mom
        Dad
sometimes late
at night
with the
sundown,
circle moon,
comets,
I relive the past
I reread this book
I watch my art
I see all of us in
each piece
we are this
expression
we are expressing
ourselves
the art that fights
        the pull of
        entropy
        a miracle
        for ~~me~~
        ~~you~~
        ~~dad~~
        ~~us~~
and we do this,
over and over,
love to love
moment to
moment

breath to breath
being to beings
        we are
and I think of
these 20 pictures
all of me
all at a distance
all of us
jewels
and I look across
our world
and I lift my
hands
and collapse the
        chasm
and I stand next
        to you
        and Dad
        jewels
and we reflect
everything
        together
20 pictures of me
        then
all at a distance
a distance
moment to
moment
we are
overcoming
healing

together.

Heidegger believes that art is the way to truth, what I have been calling Knowing. Knowing is the unconcealment of Being that opens new orientations, moment to moment. To stop resisting, shift orientations, and move with and within flow and not against.

<<Hot summer, July sun
Expansive beach
Elliot and Mary sifting sand
    me: laying out our beach towels
    catching in my legs, wind blowing
try again
    slapping in my legs
turn around, reorient
    Wind lifts, towel moving *with* the wind,   not against
    lay flat
    now we play>>

Art creates space for spaciousness, invites in the abyss, and fells a clearing for a being to enter into *the open.* In this space, you can heal. This is to *grow closer* to Being through abyssal exchange, overlapping connections. Maybe like Indra's Net or a mycelium network in an old-growth forest in the Pacific Northwest.

To come to Know yourself.

WORLD:

An artwork creates a world, encompassing you like the ocean of the biosphere, the void between the Earth and the Sun, and the Sun and all of everything. It creates space for spaciousness that is an invitation to enter into a shared experience. The world of an artwork can hold multiple beings, who were once lost in their individual *Umwelts*,   revealing them to each other,   bare, witnessing, now binding them,   unconcealing their infinite connections and reflections, creating a shared altered state of consciousness where they can learn collective ways of   Being.

EARTH:

This world has spaciousness that sets forth an earth that shelters. The earth of an artwork is the structure of the world, the ground to stand on—the physics, materials, quality of light, motion, tone, timbre, echo, harmony, order, soil, sky, sun, moon. The earth is what your toes sink into and fills our lungs with a giving origin in breath.

breathe in
breathe out

And between this world and earth, a *strife* forms and this is where truth can be won: Knowing. This Knowing is not some permanently raised curtain, but moments of

ecstasy and revelation,

taking pleasure in the unfolding strife. *A revelation that can only be known in its unfolding.*

The world of an artwork is an opening, a clearing, a free region to inhabit, flow, spaciousness; while the earth fills it with new orientations, possibilities, and hope. This clearing between the world and earth is the open, our ancestral home, full of heaven and hell, the entirety of everything, a shared expanse before Being.

But as one is unconcealed and experienced the other conceals and withdraws. For if all were unconcealed then there would be no strife, no truth to be won, nothing to Know. Just as vision needs light and dark: contrast; so we need this strife. And as we attune to the world, spaciousness and flow, so we fall out of the earth upon which we stand and sink. And when we attune to the earth and feel its warmth and shelter, we lose the world and collapse to sensation. This gradient is the strife, and through strife we come to Know ourselves.

I have sensed this in moments of creating. Losing myself, beholden to visions, that tingling sensation of dissolving in Being: waking. Glimpses at visions that, with enough luck, I can survey, move around in, inhabit, test its earth between my fingers, breathe in the air, acidic, sweet, everything.

I make gestures.

On the computer, through the camera, on the canvas, on the page, or simply Be, sensing the sensations, reorienting, creating myself to become nobody.

The world of an artwork is limitless. It isn't bound by the emergent properties of consciousness: space and time. But it is *everywhere* and *everywhen*. No boundaries. Just sensations of the natural flow. Maybe our Buddha Nature, maybe the Tao, or Dreamtime, or God, there are many names. The river of flow that sweeps you into becoming, not thinking about the past or projecting into the future, hallucinations, but simply

Becoming. *Present to the unfolding.*

When you create or perceive an artwork you found a Charon, you are transported, just don't resist, *fall*, for if you do there is actually nothing to lose, but everything to experience: Being.

The throes of creation is a Charon.
Creation is a coin ;; whether an artwork or yourself ::
to cross the river
portal <event horizon>
into the open.

Lingering sensation
Cold, cold Alberta   harder than hard
Dreaming of warmth,   maybe too warm,   the kind that blisters
your skin
and constricts
your eyes
desert, THE desert
November 9, 2019
Conference, University of California Irvine, few hours from Joshua Tree National Park
sensations of the sacred. Shamans, peyote, UFOs, secret military,
leaving LA, long road, down to one lane through a crack in a mountain
wind farms, sand and rock turning to yellow and red
into the San Andreas Fault, hyperobject quaking in my Being

BLUE SKY, WARM GROUND.
Sign: to the right desert cities
to the left *NOTHING*
Okay, I turn left

Welcome to Twentynine Palms, California
motel
hot, hot day

drive into Joshua Tree like I'm driving onto the moon.

NO CELL SERVICE. No map

breathe   in
out   drive ahead

Stop every few minutes, walk and take videos.
looking through the viewfinder with one eye closed,
experiencing only through the camera.
Ground sizzles. Maybe a snake.
Thorns on everything.

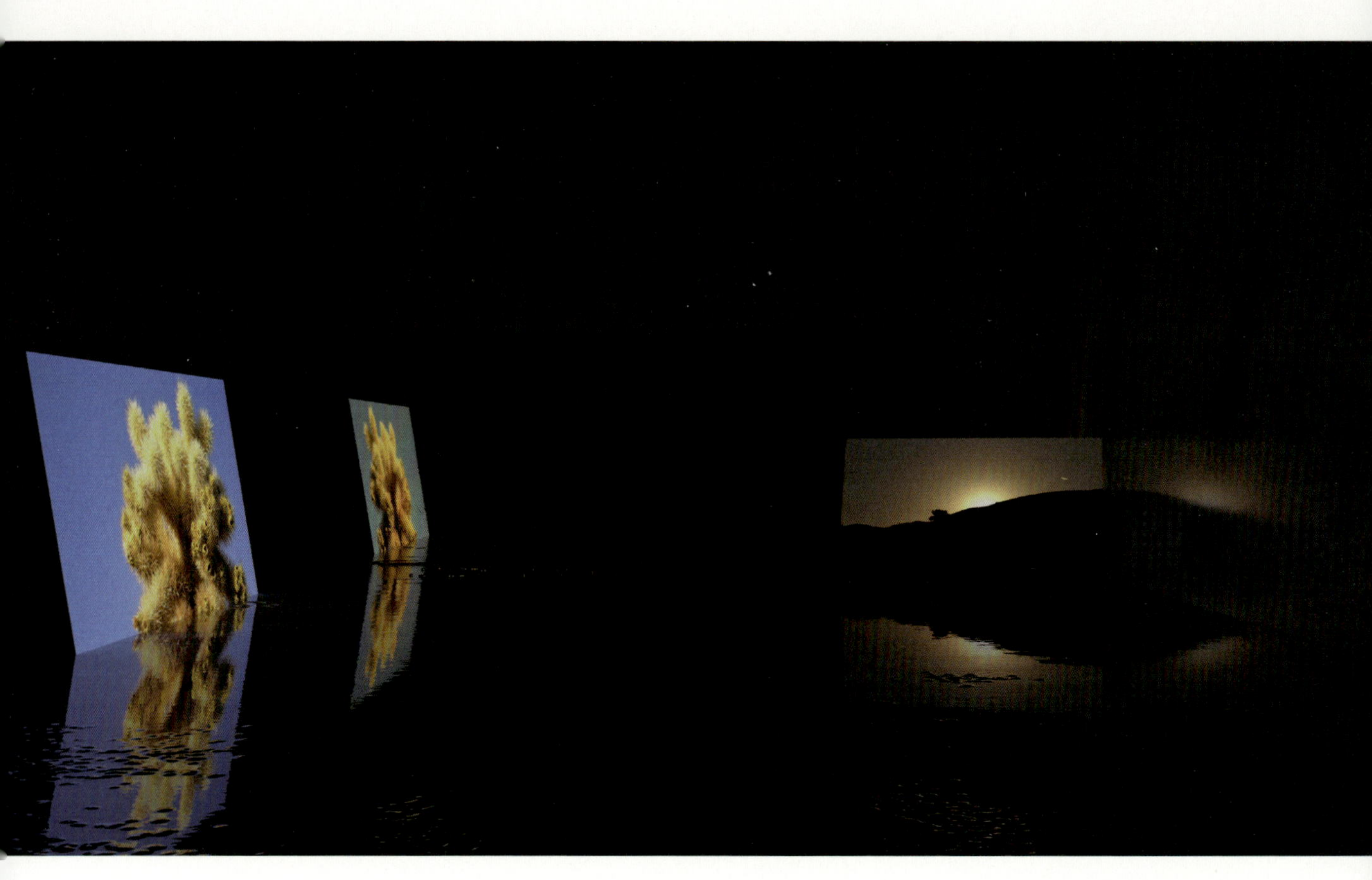

Joshua Tree and All of Everything, 2019–2020. 25-minute film created with Gary James Joynes.

Nowhere to go, so I just follow the unfolding road, the yellow ground, and the blue sky
fields of Joshua trees, hollow crisp grass, boulders dropped by god
great valleys stretching my imagination.
Come to a field. Strange cacti standing there like a congregation before god.
Sun setting. Shadows falling, I catch light through the needles. Halo
I stand and mediate as I watch the sun drop

breathe in
breathe out
breathe in   out
in   out
in

Holy Sun
Holy mountains made of the rumbling Earth, magnificent piles of rock and Time
Holy cacti, somehow living on the moon.
Sweet air, cool breeze, sound of desert, hiss
I turn and can see for miles. I see where no one can go. Mountain range leading to the
        Mojave Desert. I don't need to read the sign.
    Turn back
        Father Sun
            Mountain ghost, me
            Holy trinity
Sun bloom touching the mountain
I pull out my camera, close one eye, and watch it set through the viewfinder.
    Don't stare into the sun
    No. I'm okay
    Something happens to me that I don't yet understand.
    Some kind of changing of the guard.
    I don't live my life the same after that.

Art is essential to human experience: *humans expressing, life expressing, the universe expressing and unfolding, moment to moment, breath to breath, being to being*. The kind of art I am discussing in this book, visionary art, offers a specific disposition to creating, exploring, and Being. Visionary art is not so much a subcategory of art as it is its own impulse, its own expressing essence. Visionary art is a journey down ,,,

down into the abyss, slipping into the open, *with and within Being*, and might never amount to anything that looks like art, or to anything physical at all. It could be a sensation running up your spine, making your hair stand on end, blistering your eyes, and collapsing your sense of Self, with life and death hung in the room, revelation. I doubt it will elicit beauty, it isn't meant to, instead, placing the abyss before you, full of heaven and hell, to reorient you to Being—to enter into the flow of becoming: flux and merging. Comfort comes when you stop resisting and just fall.

And so we will fall.

Visionary art is a vital part of being human. It is our inheritance, our history, our expressing essence to enter into the pure space of the open—*a being before and within Being*.

Life is a spontaneous unfolding expression and so is visionary art. It is part of how we come to Know ourselves as living beings—*how life comes to Know itself, how the universe comes to Know itself: Knowing*. Visionary art is an eternal part of human existence and is there for everyone.

This is how we orient ourselves to *Being*
alignment
—our place in it all.

Consciousness, life, cosmos, eternity, infinity, connection.

Visionary art maps the abyss, *the inner universe.* Maps on maps, confounding, expansive, flux, black holes, empty, emptied, emptiness, surging with beings, flowing. It is an expression that makes your hair stand on end, that takes the ordinary and makes it extra-ordinary, that elevates the everyday into the sacred, that teaches and gives and connects. It is the birth of new Worlds from breath to breath, being to being:

becoming.

To Know is to have unconcealed Being. Not think, believe, or hope, but to plainly, simply, Know. But this isn't a permanent seat with Being, but ecstatic glimpses into the pure space of the open.

Reverence. Blinding. Witnessing.

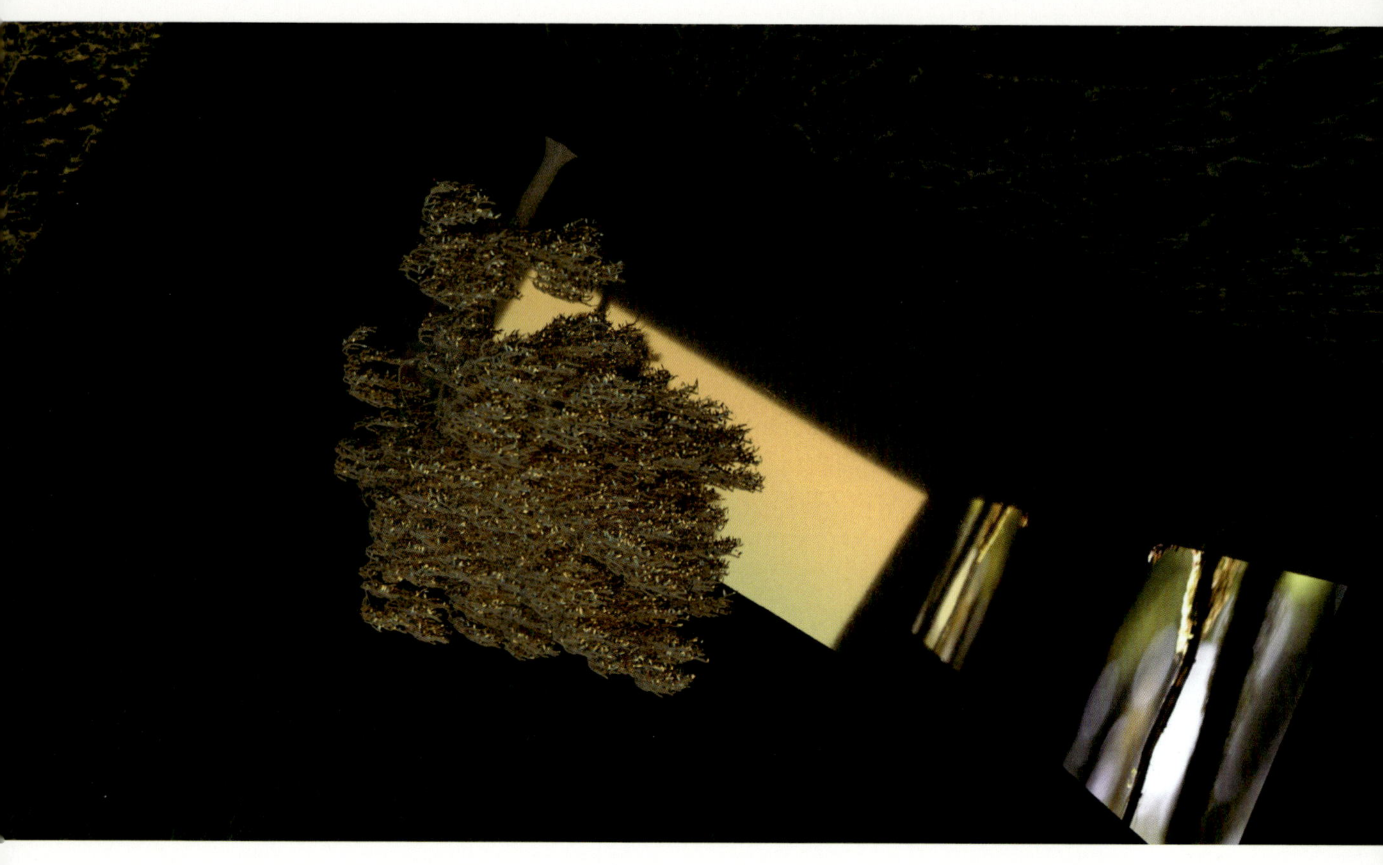

Avatar's Dream, 2021.
25-minute film co-created with Gary James Joynes and Brian Webb.

To flow in and out and between, not held. Visionary art is a way to Knowing—from one breath to the next, one being to the next. It is field recordings of a confrontation, of a relationship to the abyss within: exchange. These are never-complete sketches with still moving parts and contradictions, vulnerabilities across the whole, that do not comfort but confront, and cause you to discard the Self and fall.

Falling into the open, because falling is easier than resisting, and so we fall,
Merging

Some hold onto the waking hallucination of life and death, of the roiling river between them. And others go deep into it; they fall into terrifying places because *falling is easier than resisting*, and they take on ecstatic revelations, dissolving, merging, becoming a column of air, becoming nobody. To become nobody, you *remove* yourself, your ego, your sense that you are distinct, separate, individual. *This* is the greatest expression of self-creation: to be *reborn* as *no-one, as no-body,* as *no-thing*. Find your Charon, your ferryman, your psychopomp —

✳visions✳madness✳psychedelics✳meditation✳

— and cross the River Styx; bend down and drink from the River Lethe, forgetting the hallucinations of World and Self; slip past the event horizon,

where all directions are

down,

and merge into something larger: into the *abyssal expanse* that is both *within* and *without*, the singularity that sparks the birth of a new universe.

We go on this journey, to bear witness, to disintegrate in the flux and yet still record moving sketches outside of time or space, sketches of *Being.*

This is the visionary artist.

The abyss can hardly be described, and certainly not in its totality. *Ineffable*: it is nonrational, nonlinguistic, nonlinear, flickering with layered meanings, in flux, and always on the verge of disintegration. But so is the visionary artist. They are a conduit of thin places, of zones between this realm and the next. This has always been their role.

I feel the world in pain and now we need visionary artists more than ever, to face the abyss, to lay with life and death, and to reorient us to Being, to personally and collectively enter a state of becoming. To be reborn, to find the *origin*. To reorient ourselves towards that origin: *alignment*.

For the visionary artist, art is
field notes,
stories otherwise of this abyssal space,
reorientations to Being,
lifting the veil of hallucination,
sensing sensations,
slipping, and
sharing blistered skin and constricted eyes from the pure space of the open:

BEING

Visionary artworks are the psychological and spiritual remnants of this abyssal exploration, confrontation, and exchange, remnants that induce altered states of consciousness, a plasticity towards everything, an openness—terrified, loving—that can orient us to Being, that unconceals more than it conceals—personally, collectively, spiritually.

Visionary artists are
mystics
seers
healers.

November 17, 2020: feeling hopeful,

in the face of the great second wave of COVID, looking out over the Pacific hiding from a tsunami, my eyes part the clouds and wait for a gamma-ray burst from ancient galaxies, reading and reading the news of altered realities, stolen elections, breathing the breath under threat, coughing, asthma, watching for positive feedback loops that will turn us into Venus. But then I talk with aAron and Alice Major, poet, on Zoom.

aAron's hair is getting longer and so is mine. And both our beards are white on the chin. We talk about all of these pressing concerns. We are telling Alice about a collective aAron and I have been daydreaming about since the day we met in 2019: Distant Early Warning. He reads Marshall McLuhan's words:

// I think of art, at its most significant, as a DEW line, a Distant Early Warning system that can always be relied on to tell the old culture what is beginning to happen to it //

We came together to talk about climate change, but instead we talk about splintering realities,

and here rests in the root of the root
complete lonely islands
no portals between our *Umwelts*/worlds
nothing connecting us on Indra's Net
no reflections, just pain in all directions
scuffed and no one. shattered.

We are watching this come to a head in America right now.

So much of me experiences anger, frustration, loss, *screaming at imaginary Beings,*

beating my hands on phantom walls, breathing in hollow apparitions, empty, emptied, emptiness,

looking into the void, waiting for visions, ILLUMINATION,

hope, anything.

How do we negotiate reality now?

Distinctions where there are no distinctions?
So many us vs thems. Right // left, no, I'm looking for up // down
I'm looking to be as close to the ground, to Mother Earth, as possible for my root of the root.

aAron changed my spiritLine today when he said:
where do we begin to negotiate a shared reality?
maybe we both look out at a tree.
He says: do you see that bird?
I say: yes, I see that bird.
He says: okay. Let's both look at that bird and share it for a while.

This is the beginning of Distant Early Warning. This is part of visionary art in the twenty-first century. This is how art changes the world. This is how the negotiation begins. Erecting Worlds, creating ferries between lost islands. Portals into different universes

Of ~~you~~ or ~~me~~, or crumpled abyss,
sharing a breath together as we share a bird,
sitting in the Bodhi tree, the Being of Being.
Okay. Now let's look at something else and share that together.
Maybe this time our breath, we all share a breath.
So we continue to share experiences and a bridge forms that can be traversed
back and forth,
breathe in and out
back and forth,
breath in and out
back and forth.
breathe in and out
Mental tissue spreads. Over to there, now over to here,
then they start to overlap. connection / spirit
We start to look like a mycelial network on Indra's Net. No distinctions between me and
you, but
one.
Visionary art creates a World for us to inhabit. To leave our lonely islands, and enter into a shared World. I look across this World and I see you. The World creates space for spaciousness: invitation. Then I look at the Earth,
feel the sand between my toes,
look at the sky, blue, bluer than normal, like the sky above Mystic Beach,
warm warm sun, sheltering magnetic field,
the air in harmony with my breath,
in and out,
love,
as I look to you, across the chasm, but
this is the World of an artwork, the realm of imagination, fantasy
so I lift my hands and collapse the chasm, and stand next to you,
we look out at the expanse,
we share this moment,
this moment within the visionary artwork.

With each artwork, we draw a DEW line in that moment, then in the next, negotiation,

breath to breath, moment to moment, being to being *we are together*.

Minn shows me an image of the mask used to pin patients in place for
radiation
treatment |:|

Horror.
But also beauty, in this sculpted form. Like a fitted web.
I feel claustrophobic.
Poor faces. Hit by gamma rays.

July 2016: artists go to the Institute for Reconstructive Sciences in Medicine in Edmonton. I meet so many artists rebuilding people's faces. I meet designers working with doctors on equipment that fills me with hope. People are rebuilding dignity here.

I feel wounded by all this sensation. I walk and take pictures.
cheeks eyes nose ear

We all take turns with the haptic feedback surgery device, cutting into the digital skull, feeling the push back of the knife as it grinds through bone. O god, the sensations!

At home: I set up a greenscreen, pinning it to the wall. I set up the camera. I walk back and forth until I get myself in the composition.

Record: I start to move, nothing planned, just witnessing the movements unfold.

Spontaneous.

I bring the video to my computer, open Adobe After Effects, and start cutting, like at the Institute, an eye, cheek, lips, forehead.

I offset the timing and watch it play back.

Mid-July 2016: stuffy seminar room. Not big enough for all of us. Most of the original group from the image theatre workshop are there. The artists are presenting their initial work to the patients: feedback.

My turn: projection on screen of my mouse jumping around my desktop. Nervous. I don't feel like I can talk.

I look to Minn for confidence. Will I hurt these people? Is that okay?
I show them the lightbox image.
Patient flips his head to me.
silence
I have no idea what is to come from this exchange.
he says: *this is my violence. This is what I experienced.*
connection

Now, confidence.

I show them the video of me. Restlessly moving, never straying too far, reconnecting in unexpected, unsatisfying ways.

Patient:

this is me. This is my reality.

I now sense trust, trust to tell tough stories, stories we don't always want to hear. Stories that aren't my own, but handed to me like a jewel. About what it is like to live with this disease, to live with the disease, a disease.

A patient tells me how they just removed part of a bone from her arm to put in her jaw.

Sensations.

April 2018.
Art show: White Water Gallery, North Bay, Ontario.

Just got back from Buenos Aires a week ago. Writing most of the play *Alberta #4* after being inspired by Natalie. Mind still in the warm warm air, cafes, strange taxis, and lost in imaginary psychiatric hospitals with phantom illnesses and fictional memories.

Flight delayed, land in Toronto, running to the next terminal, jump into a propeller plane that would bring me up and up.

I walk into the airport, barely an airport, and wait forty minutes for a taxi.

I walk down Main Street and see parts of the frozen Lake Nipissing. I eat supper and have a couple of old-fashions. Dissolving into my seat.

I walk outside, snow falling and

falling.

A wet snow, like clouds that puff and puff, rest on me, collecting across time. And so I walk with all this snow on the top of my head and on my shoulders.

I step into the gallery and am greeted. Nice people. I see my work for the first time. We hung it on FaceTime a few weeks before.

Four new works: 3D-rendered images from the *Otherwise* series. I made them over January before Argentina. I barely understood the software, stumbling my way through discoveries, but it kept my beginner's mind. Everything feels like a revelation with Jeff Wall's rooms radiating in my mind. *Insomnia* and *Morning Cleaning* always resonate with me.

Then, two TVs with the cancer patients on them.

Nice opening, friendly people coming out on a night that would snow-in anyone else.

Afterwards, I find my way to a bar with live music and continue to dissolve.

The next day: artist talk.

I screen a rough cut of *Alberta #3*.

I wouldn't be happy with the piece until Kyle, aAron, and I got a shot in the rain:

June 2020.

It hurts me to watch that piece.

I think back to writing it.

Hotel room: Arizona.

Day before my presentation, the last day of the conference.

Conference theme: Time. And so I thought about time.

Start beside the pool, but my mind turns to the field notes on my computer.

hotel room dissolves no lights, shades drawn

halo of sun peeking through, hot hot day, mind slipping

scanning old field notes, luckily transcribed earlier in the year

feeling the feeling of feelings my family, my mania, Derek, Luanna

(I collapse Derek and Luanna together)

—all at once everywhen

I have been sensing something for a long time ;;something long in the making

today, I want to think through those who came before me and after me.

—about family, heredity, and legacy

I want to tell you a series of stories, not temporarily in order, about some experiences with time I've had

grabbing notes, adjusting them a bit leaving most alone

but everything was smooth, I wasn't

t

here

before, art was like one foot in front of another, a march.

this was a river

sliding and winding, with no real beginning and no real end:

absolute flow

I have never experienced this before

everything fell into place, exactly the place it needed to be

HOT FURNACE, VENTING EXHAUST

I express a story I've been waiting to hear, longing to hear to feel it all together

long and vast, much closer to the ground than I ever thought I could be

about all the illnesses that have marked my life

I read it the next day to an audience. People come up and hug me and touch me. After experiencing that reading, I couldn't attend the keynote so Maria Whiteman,

my MFA supervisor,

the kind of teacher that shows you when to use knowledge and when to wait,

like an insect waits, then you pounce,

took me out for a beer. Block up those synaptic clefts. Mute these sensations. I didn't know how concealing that was yet.

Back in North Bay:

after the film, I leave behind the traditional artist talk and we sit in a circle.

|learning from my Indigenous family|

In the middle a child, maybe eight, is moving about and drawing on a large piece of paper spread across the floor.

today, we are going to talk about trauma.

I wait.

What is going to happen?

Electric potential lifts all the hairs on our arms. We all start talking.

They talk about their old psychiatric hospital and all the art that was created there.

They talk about history and community.

A space has been created, vulnerable and inclusive, and we are all invited in.

A World and an Earth.

I redirect the conversation back to trauma. So much hurt in this town. A year ago, I learn that from the kids at CAMH who came from this town.

The person on my left speaks.

She speaks about an abusive relationship, her child looks up from the floor.

She speaks with confidence.

She says how, as you tell these stories over and over again, to friends or in therapy, that they move from being an emotional account to a series of facts. Hollow.

She said trauma isn't something outside of you but something you combat inside, something you confront, a strife. *Through strife we come to KNOW.*

I am caught by this, and it slips past my skin and finds its way into my marrow.

She finishes and she slips from behind her eyes. Others start talking. Her, motionless.

Later: she stands up and leaves the gallery. She vomits in the street.

The gallery director leans towards me and whispers:

That is her bodily reaction to this trauma.

She then gets up and leaves to help her.

I won't remember anything after that.

Donna Haraway, again, I am thinking with you. I am thinking of how unthinkable stories can literally lead us to stop thinking. How we aren't able to think with them anymore.

Then, I read Susan Sontag's *Illness as Metaphor* and see, again, how important stories are. All the war metaphors we were using at the image theatre workshop.

Natalie Loveless: *// Stories are powerful. The stories that we believe, the stories that we live into shape our daily practices, from moment to moment. They have the power to promise some futures and conceal others. They encourage us to see some things and not others //*

Thomas King: want a different *world?* Tell a different story.

In 2016, I am beginning to sense how cancer has become unthinkable. There are stories of the *disease*, the metastatic instance manifesting the cancerous body. Where will it go now:

growth ✳ recovery ✳ remission ✳ death

Then there are stories of the *illness*, the lived time spent with the disease. There is an art to doing-cancer. Maybe all those war metaphors aren't usable to think with anymore. Maybe we need to tell a new *cancer story.* After all, cures are hard to find and we are simply left with treatments.

If we don't have cancer then we know someone that does.
We feel our bodies,
we monitor the carcinogens in our diets and environments,
antioxidants!
We visit our doctor,
tests,
all to sidestep this indifferent disease.
The disease is indifferent, it strikes, it takes, but the illness is intensely meaningful.
Arguably: it is so terrifying because it provokes so many meaningful events:
doctor's office,
diagnosis,
(dizzy, dizzy, dizzy, falling to the floor,)
difficult discussions with loved ones,
their pain,
a sense of shame that you did something to make this happen,
symptoms,
treatments,
waiting rooms,

side effects,
preparing for death,
last breath,
and physically dying.
Cancer is a—species—meaning—making—event—.
It is an ancient space we all inhabit.

Nested   down   and   down
life growing   changing   flowing   replica
genetic strands   UV light   toxins   or   just change
step off the still riverbank,   sense the river flowing and flowing
can you feel the moisture hanging in the air cooling your skin?
can you feel the rush of the water at your toes, going and going?

breathe in
breathe out

the stillness of the riverbank, swatting mosquitoes looking for life, is not what incarnation
is for
fall into the water, sense the flow, breath to breath, moment to moment, being to being

okay
I fall
I've been thinking about water
feeling it crest at my feet
watching it rage in front of me
being in it
essence: flow   eons of flow
flow from some far off world,   flung into space,   time,   distance
outside mind,
comets hitting the Earth,   bathing it in water.
boiling, then liquid, air
how flow passes around you but is ~~you~~
I am a river
not a molecule—separate, unique—but the flow of all water
all at once
curving   cutting the terrain
collecting silt   eroding rocks   sometimes
raging
full
white rapids,

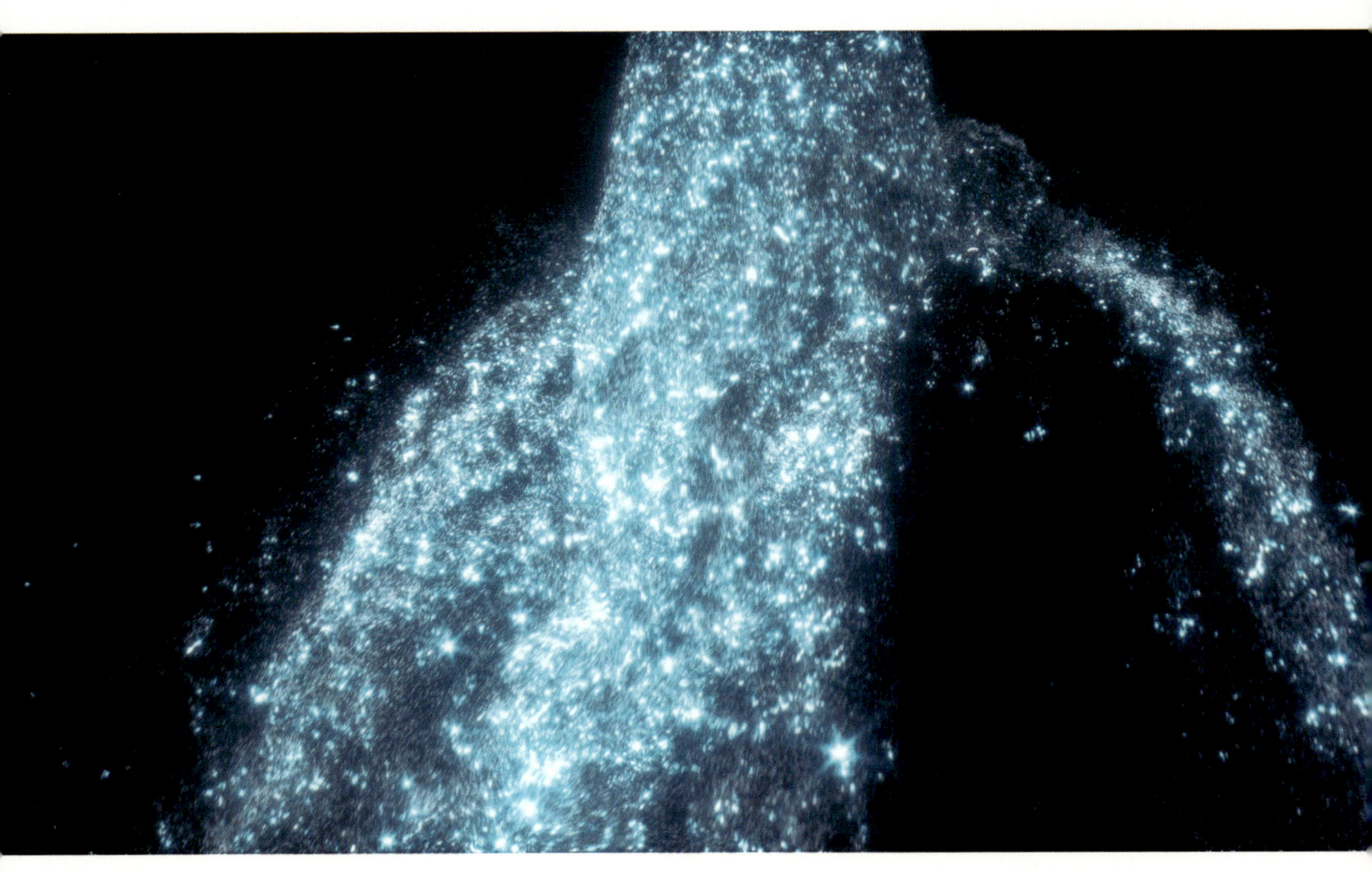

Kingdom of Illumination (jewels), 2019. 17-minute video created with Gary James Joynes.

and times of drought and ages of stillness
I breathe in an ocean into my lungs, that flows through my veins
and out my mouth and into yours
we are the same river
we twin or fork, fall off cliffs
enter into the open ocean, or
get trapped on the top of a mountain, or fall deep into the ground
and collect across time

I am the flow of light
vibration
and pushing and pulling
that streams in my mind and
out of my mind and
onto the page or
across digital time and
back into my eyes
where I meditate on the essence of flow and
time and
waiting
doing and
watching
loving
aching
I flow through time on all of this and then I am time, not locked in
a memory
ever blasting
into the future
I attune to time and time attunes to me as we slide and wind
cutting and splashing with no real beginning
and no real end

absolute flow

July 2018, before my candidacy exam, I fuse with ethologist Ellen Dissanayake's question, *What is art for?* An ethologist studies evolutionarily adaptive behaviour in beings, in this case, humans and art. She helped me see past the art-as-*thing* story I had been trying to grow out of. Her ideas dethroned art as some surplus human behaviour, something extra, and evolutionarily ground it as a normal, necessary, and adaptive human activity: *the behaviour of art.* She looks to her lived experience abroad, taking in cultural differences amongst many peoples, finding connections between art, psychological enrichment, ritual, the sacred, and spirituality. It is an act of *making-special*, to elevate an activity or thing beyond the everyday into some supra-realm of experience. Creating an altered state of consciousness superior to ordinary consciousness: // imagination, intuition,

fantasy, irrationality, illusion, make-believe, the ideal,
dream, a sacred realm, the supernatural, the
unconscious, or some other name. //

She offers seven functional ideas for what art is for:

//

1. Art echoes or reflects the natural world of which we are a part.
2. Art is therapeutic.
3. Art exercises and trains our perception of reality, it prepares us for the unfamiliar or provides a reservoir from which to draw appropriate responses to experiences that we have not been met with: flux.
4. Art helps order the world by using complex symbols to enable humans to understand and interpret, to articulate and organize, to synthesize and universalize their experience.
5. Art allows us to respond in nonhabitual ways.
6. Art provides a sense of meaning or significance or intensity to human life that cannot be gained in any other way.
7. Art allows *direct, thoughtless (or unself-conscious) experience by short-circuiting the analytic faculties. Art connects us directly to the substantial immediacy of things.*

//

This is the open.

Spring 2018: stumbling through dreamlike understanding emerging from my time learning with Natalie, she gestures to Alexis Shotwell's book *Knowing Otherwise.* Shotwell: philosopher, Professor, Carleton University.

I listen and hear:

Explicit knowing: propositional, claim-making understandings that are readily accessible within consciousness.

Implicit knowing: the background scaffolding that often goes missed as taken-for-granted ways of knowing. She articulates four types of implicit knowing:

skill-based,
socially situated embodiment,
knowing what could be in words but not currently in that form,
and *affect and feeling*.

Affect hits me. Thinking forward to something yet to happen. Arne Dietrich's universal affective content, then, still to come, Robin Carhart-Harris's psychedelic experience with links to Jung's collective unconscious. Abyssal Knowledge.

I fall back into the text.

Emotions: nameable sensations by which // beings come to know and understand themselves and their contexts, their interests and commitments, their needs and their options in securing those needs. // The named part of affective experience.

Affect: the unnameable confrontation with the unconscious, then I ache: the proto-sensory experience of witnessing the abyss. Affect is the psychic energy of the unconscious, the burned-out sensations before Being: sensations of becoming.

Affect
Those sensations that
crash to the shores
swell and overwhelm
warm and hurt
that feel like falling in a dream
that awaken me inwards
down terrified and
loving
the feeling when I start to lose my Self, falling into a VISION
beholden
awareness moving from behind my eyes and in a skull,
descending into the vision
now the eyes I look through, that strange muted colour of

dreaming with bursts of Othercolours from the Otherworld.
The fingers that grow like branches and touch and feel.
SOUND MUTED
The raging ocean of THE FEELING
You know
that one that whispers: *BEYOND HERE LIES NOTHING*
breathe in breathe out
and so, I sense that sensation, the warning signs. But they feel more
like an invitation
Okay

I use these strange eyes that aren't passively perceiving but actively
feeling outwards like echolocation. Nothing but the quantum field around
until the affective eye engages it, collapses its wave function, and
WORLD.
There is only ~~you~~ now. Without that footing in the Self, I slip
onto the changing affective sensation, holding onto nothing
flux
absolute flow and shifting awareness
open ocean
becoming
welcome home, Brad.
I weep across time
things yet to come into being
things that had come to be
hospital surgery hunger
death
pain
mind fine, body failing, child
breathe in breathe out
June 2017: mania
almost lost it ALL. SKY
body fine, mind failing
sensing that
Mary: crying, child
blistered anger
Elliot: can you open this box of cereal?, child
Candace: crying
Me: crying a decade of tears, a generation of tears, epochs
looking over the razor's edge
How far down?
I start to fall awake, jolting upwards like my heart had been
restarted. I hate myself for what I said.

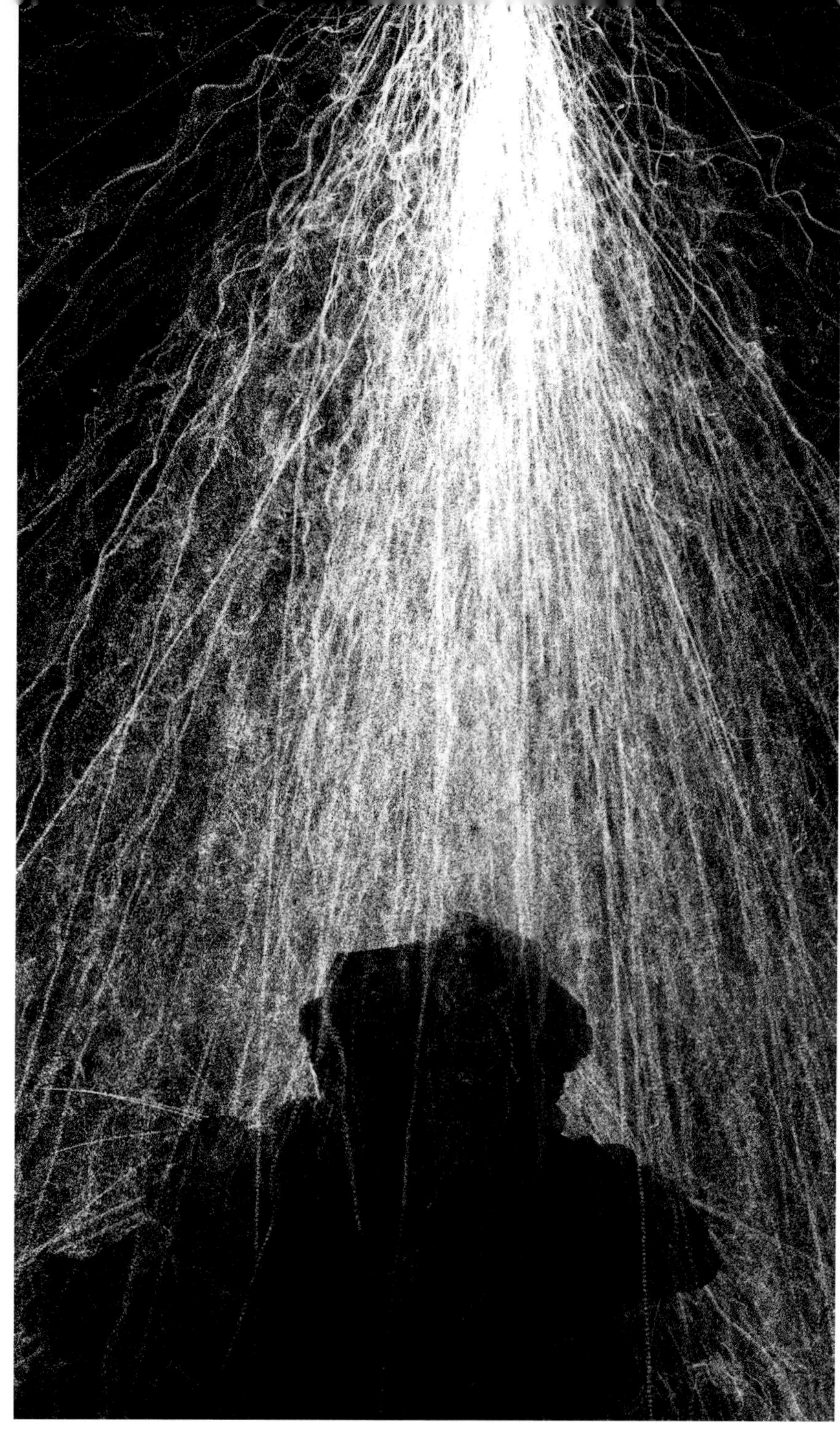

Kingdom of Illumination (God), 2021. 18-minute film created with Gary James Joynes.

Thse implicit knowledges can be cultivated towards personal and collective progress as our explicit, conscious worlds are rooted in them. To work past *unthinkable* stories and knowing. I believe visionary art is rooted in implicit ways of Knowing.

It is skill-based;
artists embody their practices;
art provides ideas before words;
and it produces, often, unspeakable affects.

Visionary art, then, is at the forefront of engaging and shaping implicit stories and Knowledges, rerooting our explicit worlds, leading to healing:

becoming.

Visionary art is *Knowing otherwise*.

The abyss is ripping, pouring, bleeding affective experience. Affect is the sensory perception of the abyss—

full of heaven and hell,
terror,
bliss,
comfort,
unmooring,
shapeshifting,
life
death.,.,.,.,.,.,.,

A visionary artwork erects a World painted with affect, sometimes the paint is nothing physical, just a sensation, revolution, blistering out in the pure space of

the open.

2018, I am dipping my toes into research-creation, full of stories and curiosity. Natalie taught me that. It ignites me to create, freely, untethered, loving and falling. After reading her manifesto I write the play *Stormshelter (Alberta #4)* in response.

Then, Owen Chapman and Kim Sawchuk, scholars, describe a subcategory of research-creation called

creation-as-research.

I don't even need to read their definition, the word alone slips past my skin and finds its way into my marrow. It rewrites my life, my work, and is a speculative account of the life that continues to unfold. This is the revolution I am looking for:

alignment.

I write autoethnographically, then, produce

Otherwise

And All of Everything

Joshua Tree

Kingdom of Illumination

The End of the World // The Birth of the World

Avatar's Dream: film ;;; now the paintings

Natalie and others explode me in an atomic blast

|||||||||||||||||||||||||||||||||||||| evaporating ||||||||||||||||||||||||||||||||||||||

as I become a column of air, a thin place, and I continue to hold onto it all these years. Maybe I could learn something more if I read all that follows, but I keep my beginner's mind, a free region of possibility, the beginning of time, the moment after particles collide in the Large Hadron Collider and unconceal the Being of the universe.

Creation-as-research was just another way to visionary art. It acknowledges the act of creation as a site of Knowledge generation. Something the visionary artist has done across time.

This is what the world needs now.

New ways to *Be.* New stories to live and breathe by. That unconceal more than they conceal. That warm and open,

ocean air
sweet
sun-kissed everything

The behaviour of art creates space for spaciousness, senses with the abyss through affects, and drops field notes as the visionary artist and the abyss exchange back
and forth.

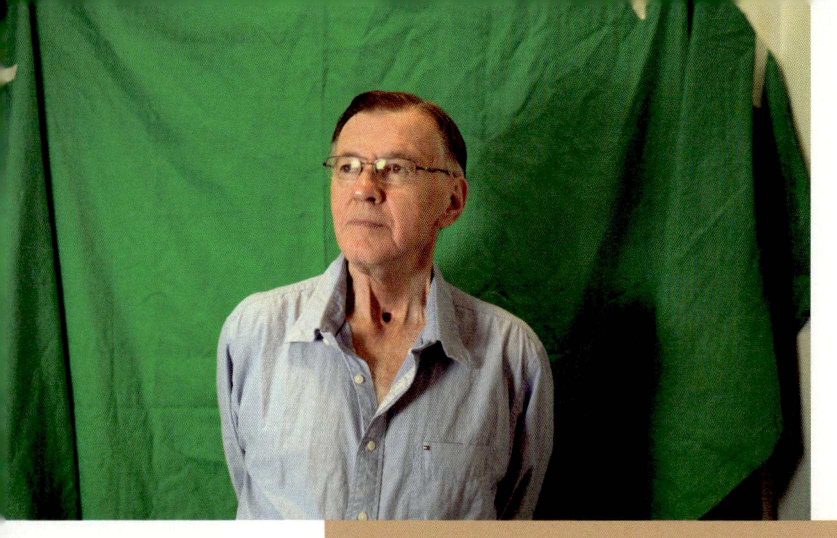

(Top) Behind the scenes with Bernie in fall 2016. (Middle) *Waiting Room*, 2016–2017. 1-minute video. (Bottom) *Waiting Room*, 2016–2017. 1-minute video.

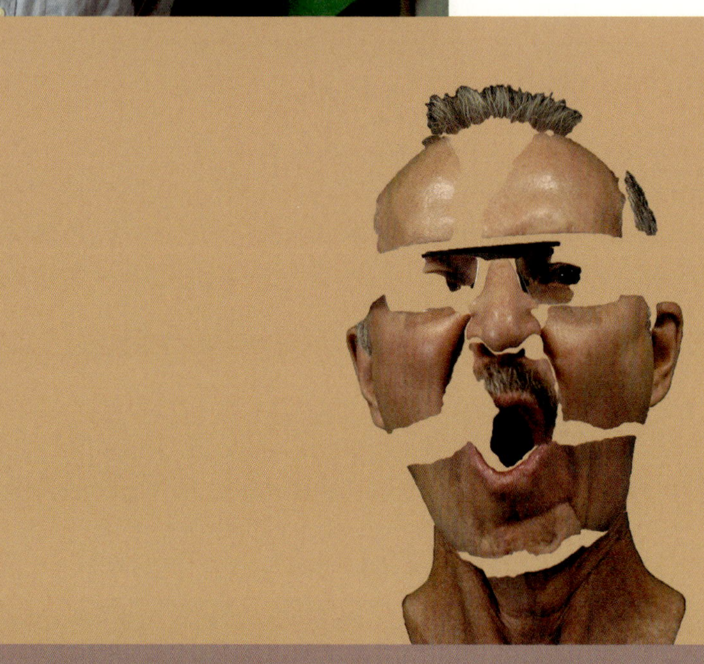

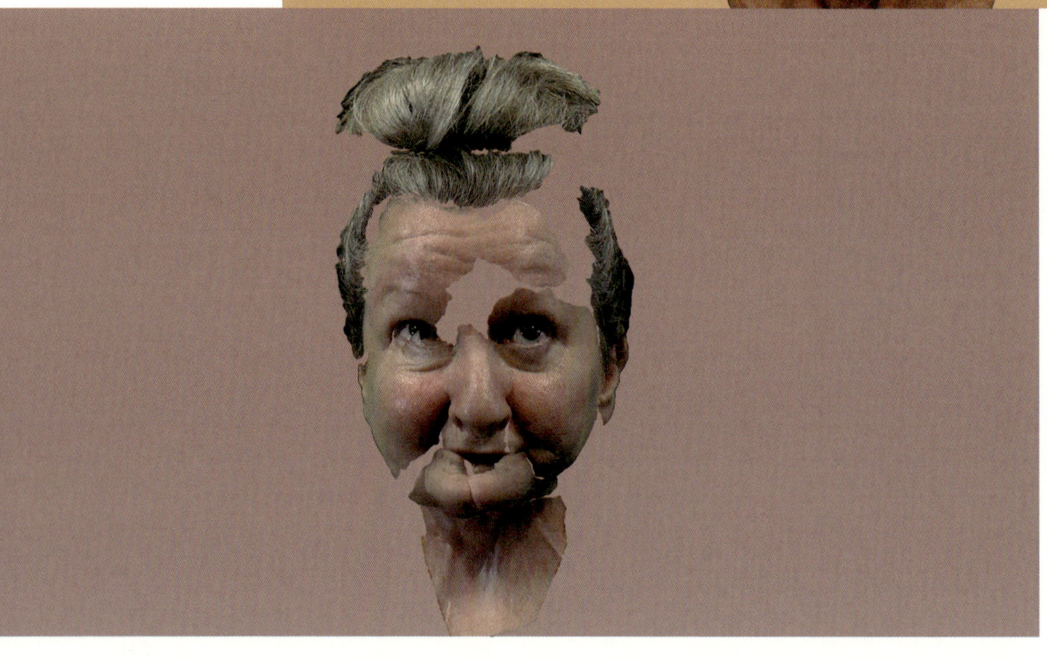

Cooling September day, 2016.

Four head and neck cancer patients, small art historian office: Lianne McTavish, intellectual, pushing me to grow back in 2012 and onwards.

I plug in the computer and monitor I brought and show them the videos I have been making of family and friends. To give them an idea of what I have in mind for today.

They want to give it a shot.

Spontaneous.

I use books on a bookshelf to pin the green screen in place. Daylight entering through the window and I set up another light to soften the shadows.

I set the camera on the tripod, set the composition, and simply press record.

I say: move ,,, move how it feels natural.

One sits and moves. She says it hurts her scars. I say to move in a way that feels open.

Everyone gets a turn.

They inspire each other.

We laugh and talk about all kinds of things.

Things everyone should say.

It takes three months,
and a computer upgrade,
but I have a video of Ken and a video of Sharon.
Then I make a few photographs.
Leslie hangs above my couch.
Bernie is etched into my marrow.
Sharon, Kim, Ken continue on my out breath.

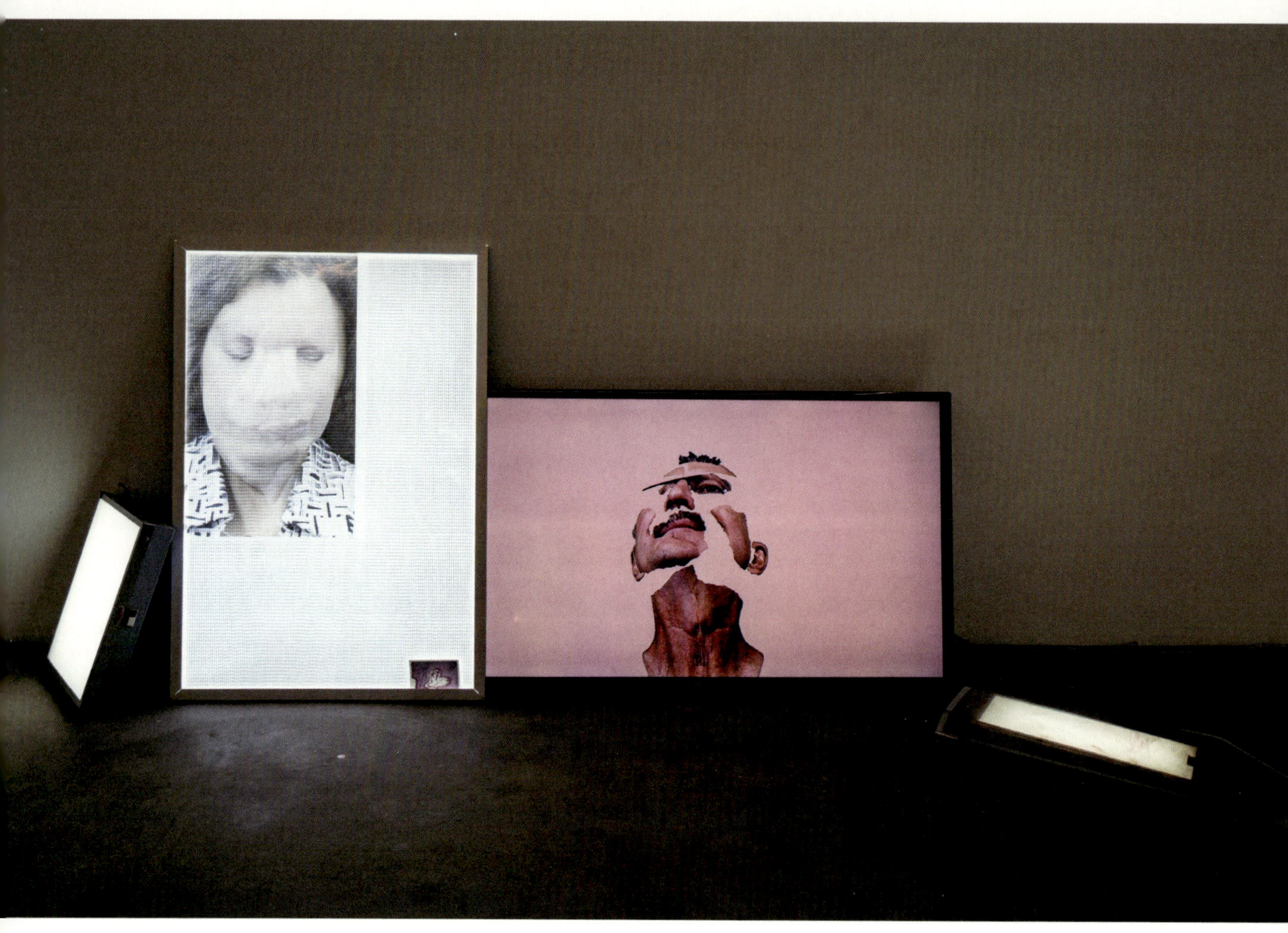

Installation, *Waiting Room*, 2017. dc3 Art Projects. Edmonton, Alberta.

We do something special today. Sure we make art, but we also make trust, *create* it. Trust to sense and feel *together*,

gaze into CANCER,

lay with death, pain, hurt, loneliness, suffering.

Story it otherwise.

October 2019: I spoke at the book launch for the publication of the project: *Art-Medicine Collaborative Practice: Transforming the Experience of Head and Neck Cancer.* Technical problems showing my slides, but I talk about telling stories, all the things I learnt from Natalie, Haraway, King, and Sontag.

Then Leslie, Ken, Kim, and Bernie stand up.

It was like they had been touched by God

|Lazarus|

They speak about the organization they started to support people with head and neck cancer. How, before this project, they struggled to work, lost their friends, family, and hurt and hurt and hurt. They speak these words and look

reborn.

Holy!

I sit and watch sensations

love connection

Yes, still pain, but also

balance

reorientation.

ALIGNMENT

Life and death hang in the room,

Hello.

Cancer is an apocalypse, it ends Worlds: a revelation that can only be Known in its unfolding.

Cancer is changing, flowing, becoming. Everything is changing, flowing, becoming:

breath to breath, the being to being *we are.*

Future: now with an end date. Terrifying. Charon is waiting.

But that is then, and really, when we really look close, all we are is NOW.

They speak to me:

Be with the surgeries. Be with the treatments.

Be with your family when everything feels normal.

Be with the pain. Be with yourself.

Be with the hugs and tears and fears.

Be with transformation!

Holy! Holy! Holy!

Be with death.

Be with everything.

Ready for *the* origin.

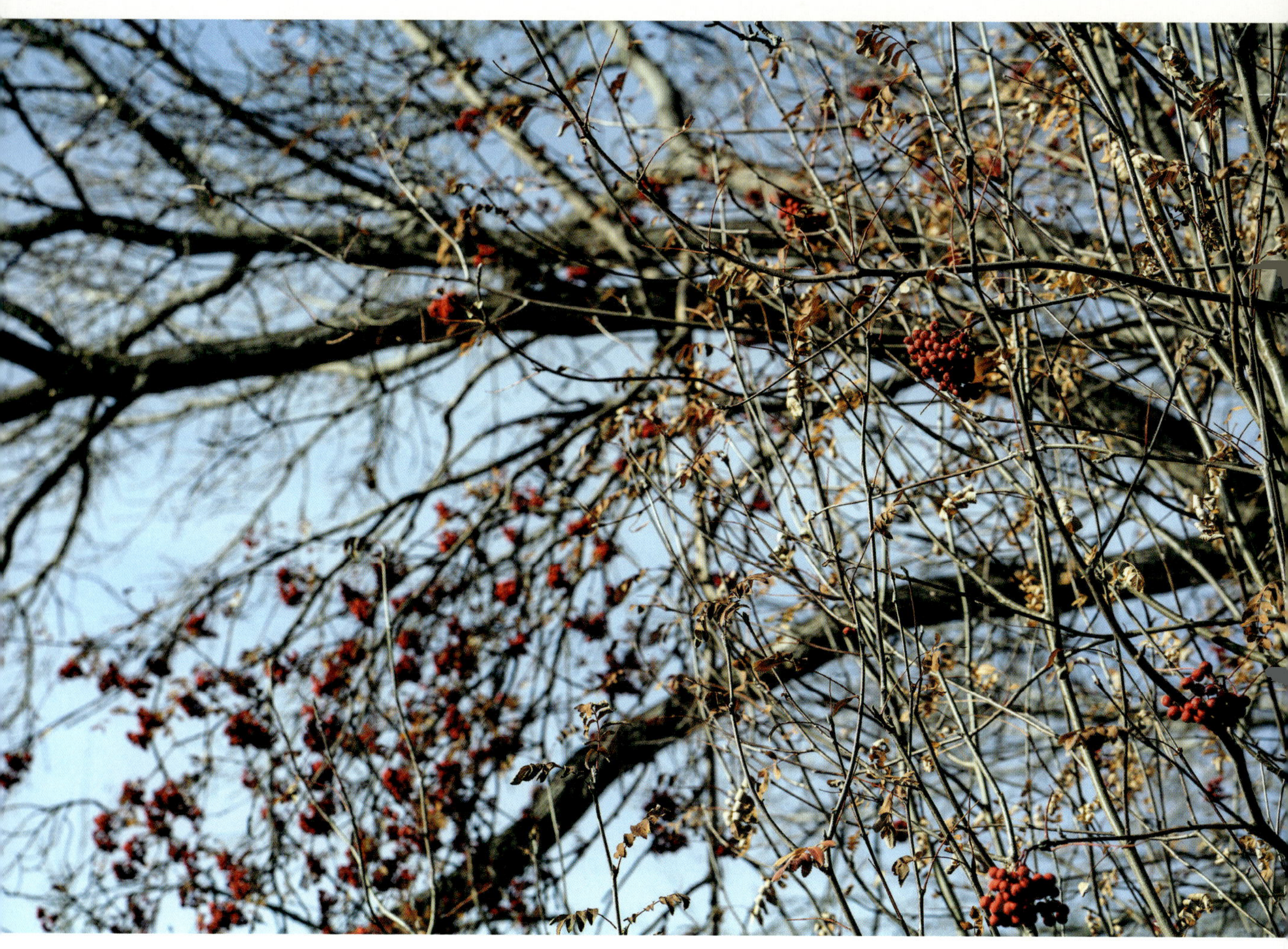

Ready to fall.

I think of you, Grandma.

New Year's Eve 2003: I am crying on Candace's shoulder in her parents' house. I feel a moment coming, an event horizon that I will pass, into a universe without you. Here I am, in this room, on Candace's shoulder, crying a deep cry of recognition of things to come.

We always have dinner at your house on Sundays. Until we move to British Columbia in July we have dinner at my parents' house every Sunday. We just had our last Sunday dinner as they left yesterday, back to Alberta, unsure when COVID will allow us to be together again.

Late October 2004: you have been going for experimental therapy for months,,, lesions forming on your arms,,, We order food in that Sunday night. All conversation, all vision from this dinner is gone, just Knowing, feeling out affectively into these memories and simply being with and within that memory.

We sit around the table I know all too well and the phone rings. You answer it. Your cancer is very advanced and you need to go to the hospital immediately. Like a tsunami we all move, dizzy, falling in our minds, in preparation to help you to the hospital. We leave that table for the last time together.

I leave to the stairs at the back entrance when I gaze back through the hall, into the dining room. The room loses form and you both disappear from vision, crossing out of my mind and into a pure space. I feel you and Grandpa going through a conversation you must have been preparing for for some time. But you are simply showing him how to take messages from the phone.

O you loved to talk on the phone

I turn my head and walk out the back door of the house and the brightness of that late October day pierces through the fading memory and I can see all the red berries on the ash tree at the back. A tree I have spent my life looking at.

I get to the hospital. I look through a pane of glass and see you in that damn hospital gown, across that damn hospital bed.

pain.

a portal opens.

===

I walk through,

===

then I walk across the room, stand across the bed from you, and burst out crying, tears of grief. You reach across the bed and we collapse into each other, whispering words that are now gone.

July 26, 2020:
I'm over here now, British Columbia.
Vancouver Island.
Victoria.
Soon Cobble Hill.
    Hopefully.

I've been witnessing the sky gradients out of mind.
Blurred moons of Jupiter.
Misting Saturn.
Circle moon.
    The open.

ALL SKY. MIRROR OCEAN. Bliss, happiness, presence, generosity.
My camera is recording right now.
Listening to "Sad-Eyed Lady of the Lowlands."

Every day is so long—wow. It's so giving and giving and warm—
        ocean flow
            and sand,
            and rock,
            and family,
    my girls and yours, too.

    It's been so long. Saying so long, Grandma; so long ago.

O god, I loved,
—love you.
But I saw your parents' graves,
    I saw your grave,
        I saw my   grave.
        Then, it happened. Speaking closely with aAron. Mid-December 2019.
        A story, one I needed to hear, then a vision and mind aligns to Being:
        I can try and wait.
        Healing.
    I see you in my girls and their sun-kissed faces
    —radiating Candace, holy Mary, golden Ellie.

I look at my dad, your son, enduring: Parkinson's, then, stroke.

This is something you look to your mom to
    —comfort.
    I gaze back to Elliot's room, then across to Mary's. Every pain we share—
    for now. I can read the signs, as the road unwinds.

I'm sitting here with Candace.
Just about to have a conversation.
Looking out in the expanse of World and Mind.
    No more blistered skin or constricted eyes.
    Dilated everything, the openness for the open.
    The pure space.
    Everything right in front of me.

February 2017: I fall back into a room at CAMH.
I lift out of the drum session. We hand back our drums and I never see the volunteer again.

Kids leave the room.

I stay seated. What am I doing here again? I slip in a daydream. Maybe a real dream.

Ruptured: young boy asks me to play chess with him.

Okay.

We talk over the game. He says he is leaving tomorrow. His mom is coming to get him.

He wins the game and I never see him again.

I walk through the unit, past the panopticon, and see a partially completed mural with a patched over, fist-sized hole. Nothing else to see. I go back into the activity room and sit, gazing out a wall of windows that looks over expensive Toronto condos.

A young man is pacing behind me, speaking intensely to himself. I am trying to assess this new space of uncertainty. I have no training to be here. Other than my own lived madness.
I try to open myself to this experience.

I say hello. No response.

I ask him his name.

Jesse. Then he walks to the other side of the room and keeps talking to himself.

I won't press him. *He is on his journey and I am on mine.*

I walk across the room and see a pile of papers that have personal messages patients have written to each other: group therapy. I found Jesse's name and read the message:

Jesse, you are my dearly cared for people ever.

FOR ELLIE

August 30, 2013.
Ellie, I remember when you were born. I saw a newborn baby. They lift you to your mother's chest and you look at each other for the first time. I see her tears of joy. I hear sounds of thunder and I look over my shoulder, out the window, looking across the prairies I know so well—illuminating the space between the raging clouds and the silent ground, igniting my imagination.

As I look at you on your mom, I have a rush of memories I haven't had yet. Like you and I have lived this life a hundred times and this was another cycle. I feel all that we will share at once.

September 15, 2020, I drop you off at school, sky like a veil, smoke from forest fires raging in the south: Washington, Oregon, California. But you are at nature school, here to forge a lifelong connection to *your home between your toes*.

Late one July summer night you wake up while I am recording the stars. It is warm, you are in your pyjamas and we go outside.

We look at Jupiter, bright, almost visible moons
closing closer to Saturn, once in 800 years
Later, Mars in opposition, on close approach, decades of waiting
Then we went out the front and found NEOWISE. Travelling on vibrations, over
billions of miles, over
billions of years, *falling*,
waiting for alignment, then,
warmth of the sun,
blue tail weeping,
coming to drop angelic
visions,
igniting your imagination,
raising the hair on your arms,
bare awareness,
curiosity's desire,
glimpsing at Being,
looking up and up across
time, again
looking for an origin.

Everything I felt at the beginning of time, I feel unfolding now, with you.

I still feel forward, moments coming as we pass breath to breath. Times for holding, times for bracing, times for celebration as you express your essence and unfold across time.

FOR HIM

February 2017: big winter storm, nurses talking about their two-hour commute through the snow, cold. I had attended group therapy yesterday with the kids and now sit alone in the activity room as they attend school in a room across from the nurses station.

Afternoon: gym. Kids get into shorts and loose shirts and I have my jeans on with a muted green sweater. Down the elevator, but they opt out of using the tunnels to get across campus to the gym and want to walk outside. The nurse says it is fine. Cold.

Once we get in the gym everyone breaks off. Some run on treadmills, others pretending to lift weights, but most go and grab basketballs, badminton rackets, and nets. A couple kids and I play basketball and we build up a sweat. Something I didn't do often yet. My clothes didn't help, but it was fun. In unimaginable circumstances we are having fun.

Too hot, I take a break. A twelve-year-old kid comes up to me and opens a side door outside and lets the cold cold air stream in like a storm. He is so young, curly hair, starting his growth spurt, just like I did at his age.

Without prompting, he starts showing me all the scars on his body:

knife wounds,
cigarette burns,
self-harm.
I feel in my mind to the scars
aching on my stomach.

He tells me about his abusive father.

He tells me about living on the streets of Ottawa.

Under a bridge, adults,   rapes.

He told me about meth and alcohol. About his twenty-one-year-old boyfriend.

I couldn't process this for anyone, let alone a child.

Elliot,   Mary,   me. Children.
Sensations venting from some unknown space.

I had nothing I could say: listen. I see that sometimes the only thing I can do is let someone tell me a story.

His movements change, he starts to twitch, his eye contact starts to break. These stories are over taking his body.

April 16, 2016.
Mary, I remember when you were born. You came so quickly they couldn't give your mom pain medications. I watch our doula and the nurse guide your mom through the most intense experience of her life. I stand here, a warmer than average April day, in the middle of the night, becoming aware to the continuum of women that unfolded into this moment. A line up of unbelievable women. A generational strength that you will have, a strength I see developing every day.

When you are born, you are blue, and they rush you to the side and two nurses begin massaging your back. I just watch your small face, then, breath. The breath to breath that you are today. They hand you to your mother and you lay on her chest. She cries as the nurses push on her stomach, but she holds you like a mother holds their newborn child.

4:00 a.m.: my parents show up and I hand you to my dad and introduce you to him:

This is Mary Necyk.

Your great-grandma's name, his mother's name. He holds you, looks at you, and cries a cry of layers.

Mary, I am looking at you right now, four-year-old Mary. You and I are one. When I am happy, you are happy. When I suffer, you suffer. You ride all the vibrations of Being with me, and the madness, the ebb and flow of bipolar, of slipping then ascending.

I am sorry.
I don't want this to hurt you, wound you in love,
but we are one,
in mirror,
fall breath to breath together,
whether exhaling a scream,
or bursting a laugh from the root of the root,
the bud of the bud,
that wants to take hold, find comfort, safety, to grow, up and up,
into the sky of the sky, becoming the tree of life,
your origin.

O Mary, my Mary.
This is the first time we have done this together.
The first time around.
I look into your eyes, and you look into mine.
I lift my imaginary hand and wave,
hello in there.

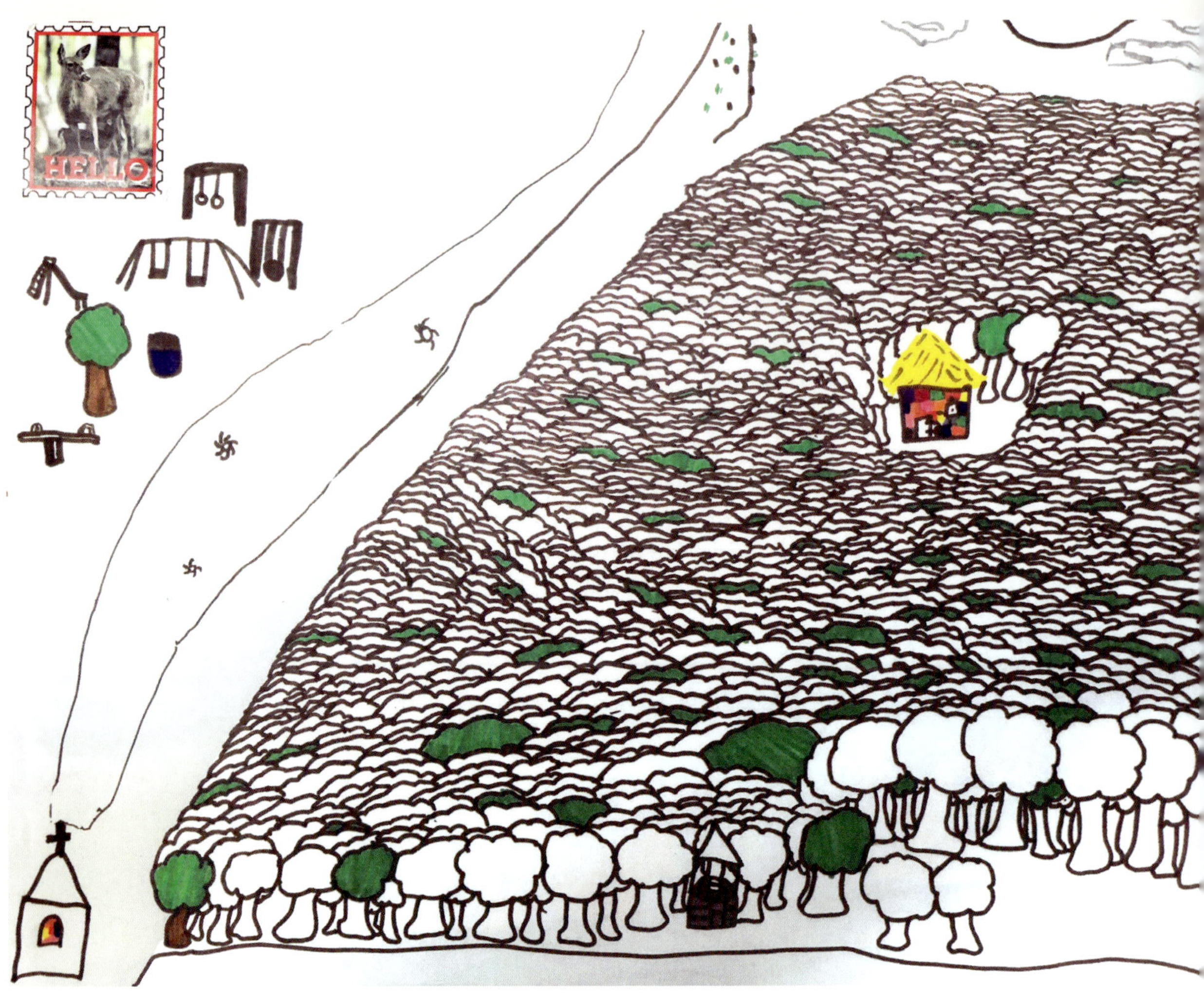

1991. My seven-year-old drawing, electrified and illuminated deep in the forest.

Second day in 2017: it seems like everyone left, but Jesse, and a unit's worth of new patients were admitted. When I came through the door I felt like I was admitted. I look at the locked doors, then to the panopticon, nurses breathing and fogging the windows of the mind, and I wonder if they will listen to my request to leave: if this gets too tough. It's a sensation I don't understand yet.

I sit in the activity room and slowly the new kids start to come in. I say hi, but slump down in my chair, not sure what I am doing here. A fourteen-year-old girl comes in, sits next to me, and introduces herself. She is a personable kid. More confident than I was, am. She smiles and her teeth have disintegrated. It makes my teeth ache, sending signals to nerves across my body. I want to give this girl a hug, like I would Elliot after a bad dream. This is a bad dream.

I tell her I am an artist and I am doing some research at the hospital. She thinks that was pretty cool.

would you like to make some art with me later?

okay.

The kids are making small chat, but it feels like they are sizing each other up. How hard each of them are. I think about Elliot playing with kids at the park, each a superhero with powers better than the next kid's, and that kid is the best at the next thing. These kids talk about drugs, fights, and streets.

An adult comes in: occupational therapist. More kids follow her in. Maybe thirteen now.

I get up and introduce myself to her and she introduces me to the unit's school teacher. Everyone is warm.

I say I'm an artist and am wondering about the art supplies there.

They ask:

are you doing art therapy?

no. Research.

into what?

lived experience of mental illness and recovery.

They don't get it. I don't get it either. Yet.

They have next to no art supplies. Dried paints, broken pencils, printer paper.

Kids are getting louder. We stop talking and they ask me if I would like to sit in for this session: a form of group therapy.

They pass the broken supplies around and ask each kid to make a drawing. Kids don't need inspiration, they haven't yet forgotten they are artists. Some draw like Elliot, three, some draw like a teenager. After a bit the therapist asks them if they can share their drawings. The girl I just met turns her's to the group and says this is a drawing of my baby. He is one.

She shows her holding him, smiling.

She talks about his birth and the months he had to stay in the Hospital for Sick Children in Toronto and all his surgeries. She talks about her meth addiction and how it impacted him.

It feels like she has told this story a hundred times before and this was another round. A series of facts without emotions. But there was tenderness in her word choices and drawing. She spoke about living near North Bay. A few other kids spark up and say they are from there too. They start comparing landmarks.

The discussion continues around but I can't move past this girl. Her story.

After they leave, I look at the drawings. They are kid's drawings but the stories within these images were beyond kids' stories. I stay past dinner that night. I find it difficult to leave.

December 2015: University Hospital, Edmonton.

Year into my artist-in-residence with transplant patients at the hospital and I am in an elevator with an art therapist on our way up to the psychiatric ward. She has a pushable cart of art supplies and is warm.

She goes around the unit, inviting patients to join. One of the nurses tells me it's Bob Dylan's birthday on his son's birthday. He then points at my Dylan shirt. He shows us to a room. Small, almost like a closet, but we fit ourselves and five patients in.

I was there to simply observe, not knowing this would play into a moment I couldn't imagine happening, yet. Something larger and longer.

She lays out a large piece of paper and everyone circles around it. She hands out pens // nice pens from an art store. She says they were donated.

We all start to freely draw on the paper in the areas closest to us. Talking: small chat. But some stories get too difficult, about pain, enduring, but everyone was on different points in their journey, and some winced. The art therapist gently moves the conversation back into a safe space for everyone, moment to moment, negotiation.

Spontaneously: she reaches across the page and draws a line from one patient's drawing to hers. This is like a lightning strike that explodes potential, erecting a new World with new Earth to shelter. Everyone starts reaching across the page and expressive marks fill the page: laughing. She then turns the page clockwise and everyone starts drawing with someone else's drawing.

Some patients get tired | pills and pain | and slump back in the room or fall out into the unit. Others find their way in. Conversation fills the room.

The art therapist kept everyone together, creating space for them to express themselves, all the tough things that led to them sitting in this room, but made it safe. Redirections. This was a porous space that could be whatever each person needed at that point in their journey.

A year and a bit later: CAMH.

Earlier in the day, the unit manager and I went to an art store down the street and bought some new art supplies from some money donated by a parent.

I lay a large sheet across some combined tables in the activity room. Kids spill in, conversation, everyone cool. I don't know what will come of this but I try to channel the World the art therapist created. First, some free drawing, then lines connecting us, turn the page, conversation, energy fills the room, then tired, and kids spill off to their own ideas. With the kids left, we take some of the new markers and colour in the shapes created as we freely draw across the page. The new girl thought we should paint over the mural in the hall. Fix the punched in hole and its incomplete design.

I talk to the unit manager and she thinks it's a great idea.

We take some small rollers and I thin out the white paint and we wash it over the old mural. One kid tips over a bucket of paint, then splashes it on another kid's clothes. They laugh, which I haven't experienced with these kids, in this place, under these circumstances.

Kids being kids.

They have to stick to the schedule and have alone time in their rooms. I took the co-created drawing and pencil it onto the wall. It was simple enough to let anyone, no matter their skill level, join in and paint: little shapes for a block of colour.

An hour later, they come out of their room, grab a brush, pick a colour, and start painting. They don't need any instructions. They are all artists. They form a line along the wall, each working on an area. We talk freely over the painting filling the hall and our spirits with expansive connection. The new girl steps back and sits with me on the windowsill and we talk about all the possibilities this mural could be. We talk about the things that led her here. Unbelievable child, mother, hope.

I wish I could photograph this moment, even if just for myself to remember it clearly, put me back in that footing, behind those eyes.

I see kids being kids: laughing, telling jokes, being playful. I don't see patients with unbelievable pasts. I feel many things I don't understand yet.

Each day we work on the mural, colour by colour. I take a one-day side trip to Montreal to meet a curator and when I come back they had used their hands to make all the leaves on the trees. When I came in, they rush from the activity room to show me their progress.

We continue to work on it together but don't finish it before my trip is over. A few months later, I take the elevator up to the unit and look at the mural. It remains unfinished but it brings back a rush of memories.

A year later, I am cleaning my studio and a large piece of paper falls out. Pastel powder spills onto my floor and covers my hands as I open its folds. O kids, I forgot you made me a going away drawing. Marks everywhere, bursting with colours. It says thanks. Thanks, kids.

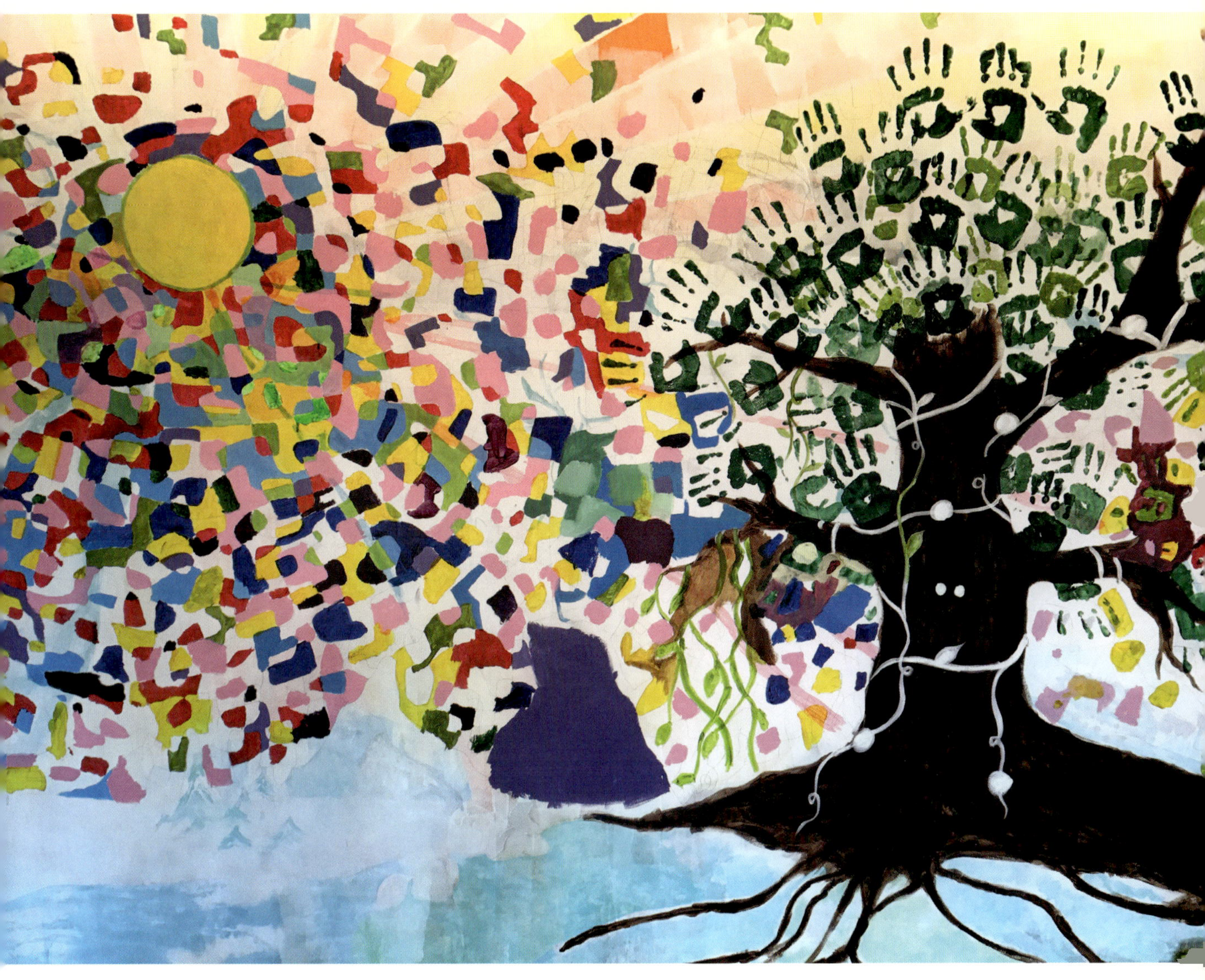

Unfinished 15-foot mural at CAMH's Youth with Concurrent Addiction Unit, February 2017.

I remember having an intestinal attack grade one
I remember playing Super Nintendo on a roll-in cart. There was a kid next to me
tubes everywhere. I was so sick. Then she died.
I finished grade one in the hospital school. Thirty years later, I'm still there.
I remember the kids there, all different ages, IV carts, tubes everywhere.
I don't know how they taught us all at different ages. Maybe more of a symbolic act.
Sometimes those are important.

Neuroscience is the practice of looking at the organ of the brain to find connections between matter and consciousness. Areas mapped for vision, motion, bodily awareness, memory, emotion, higher-level thinking, planning, acting, and so on. How these regions interact with consciousness remains the *hard problem*: how consciousness emerges from complex interactions of matter. Donald Hoffman has ideas on that.

The Default-Mode Network (DMN) has emerged as a neural network tied to a central experience of consciousness: I, your sense of Self.

The DMN is a network that connects part of your prefrontal cortex, the most evolutionarily evolved, most uniquely human part of our brain, posterior cingulate cortex and angular gyrus, the hubs for the ancient emotional and memory regions of the brain connecting our universal knowledge, our ancestral inheritance of all life on this planet to us.

The DMN turns on when we are not doing anything, your default state,
it gives us our sense of Self,
our ego,
mediating our waking-conscious experience of the world,
reality-testing.
It is the autobiographical network of our brain.
It is how we self-reflect, become Self-aware.
It is how we story.
Telling you stories that are personally relevant.
Also, it is a time machine.

It takes us back in time to ruminate on the past or projects us into the future, making connections from the past to react, for better or worse, to the uncertainties of the future.

The DMN mediates our experience of the world, constricts it, and compresses it into easily understandable stories: erecting a personal world to inhabit.

Like Heidegger, this is the region of being human that lays like a trap, keeping us from the pure space of the open. It robs us of the present and
dis-{orients}
us from Being.

While it is tremendously adaptive and crucial in humans' evolutionary success, it is potentially a physical connection to the ceasure of oneness, narrating that you are an individual, creating insides and outsides, telling you all kinds of stories of hallucinations.

// It matters what stories make worlds, and what worlds make stories. // This is the network where stories and worlds collide.

Robin Carhart-Harris:
visionary neuroscientist and dreamer,
central figure in the psychedelic renaissance, Imperial College London, now University of California San Francisco,
has proposed a theory of consciousness that describes the Default-Mode Network's effect on the brain and conscious experience. Entropy is the level of disorder within a system where higher entropy describes more disorder and lower entropy less. With the brain as the system and neural communication as ordered or disordered, Carhart-Harris proposed two modes of consciousness: primary and secondary.

He posits that the DMN lowers entropy, lessens disorder, and constrains your conscious experience to promote realism, foresight, careful reflection, and an ability to recognize and overcome wishful thinking and paranoid fantasies. It allows more precision in our thought, our ruminating, and our projections into the future. It was, for this reason, why we evolved the DMN—to better predict our future, respond to changing circumstances quickly, and, ultimately, survive.

However, to do this the DMN filters and limits conscious experience. This includes perceptions, but it also limits the possibilities of thought. As the brain's entropy has lowered, it communicates less globally and, instead, communicates to limited regions. It is a narrower, more constrained world for you to exist in. It also is how we create the boundaries of our World. *Distinctions where there are no distinctions.* He called this conscious experience, secondary consciousness. It is secondary because it evolved from a more primordial form of consciousness, what he calls primary consciousness.

He posits that this primary consciousness is closer to the consciousness, or World, our ancient ancestors would have experienced or what children experience. He studies this mode of primary consciousness through the application of psychedelics into subjects' central nervous systems.

Psilocybin is the psychoactive compound in several genera of fungi, commonly referred to as magic mushrooms: a classical psychedelic. They have been used for healing and spiritual development in Indigenous Peoples for millennia. Over the past decade, they have been part of the psychedelic renaissance in neuroscience for their psychiatric applications, but also their potential for revealing the workings of consciousness.

// They are for psychiatry, what the microscope is for biology or the telescope is for astronomy. //

Carhart-Harris posits that psilocybin increases brain entropy, dysregulating the Default-Mode Network and allowing the brain to communicate globally. It manifests primary consciousness by dissolving the ego, the sense of Self. Phenomenological accounts of psychedelic experiences report enduring death, commonly referred to as ego-death—the overwhelming clawing onto life, the Self. However, once one *dies* it isn't nothing but everything. People report a

dissolving,
merging,
then, sense of oneness,

whether they say with nature, Mother Earth, God, or universal consciousness.

They have entered the pure space of the open, *a being with and within Being.*

Psychiatric disorders, such as depression, anxiety, OCD, PTSD, and addiction are being theorized as conditions arising from an overly engaged DMN. Where the network has become too fixed and constraining one's world, turning in on itself and causing disordered consciousness—dis-{orientations} to Being. A single dose of psilocybin, amongst other psychedelics such as LSD, DMT, and MDMA, and its entropy-inducing ability have been able to clinically treat these disorders many magnitudes greater than our best pharmaceuticals and behavioural therapies. Crucial is the talk therapy before and after that helps you integrate these insights and understandings that emerge from the psychedelic experience—psychedelic-assisted psychotherapy.

Further, an active area of study for psychedelics is in end-of-life therapy as cancer patients experience depression, anxiety, and suffering heading towards death. But when these people *die* with psilocybin, they report, in numbers, that they no longer fear death and have learnt how to live. Allowing them to enter the transformation of death: present with Being.

Psilocybin and its entropy-inducing qualities have a significant impact on the personality trait of *openness to experience*. Higher openness to experience aids people in experiencing uncertain situations, enabling them to enjoy variety, beauty, art, and many of the experiences that make life worth living. It is a very prosocial personality trait. Psilocybin has been shown to have long-term, maybe lifelong effects.

From clinical trials, individuals report that their psychedelic experience was one of the most significant experiences in their lives. Right up there with falling in love, the death of a parent, or the birth of a child.

Psilocybin takes you to the abyss,
  death,
  then rebirth
shows you *a* origin, (different each time)
Wow!
and all of everything
Takes you from *here* to *there.*
Northern Star of Being,
compass:
  alignment.

And, with enough luck, it will bathe you in love. The kind that burst forth from your heart, radiation, or the painful one of *growing closer: overlapping connections.* Like the mycelial networks they came from, now in interspecies alignment with the overlapping networks of our brain, merging into consciousness :: sharing the space of consciousness with another being.

Psilocybin is a Charon, one that should be approached with reverence,
that teaches you
  how to live, *Be.*

Healing: an ecstatic transformation that can only be known in its unfolding, falling into flux as you enter into a state of becoming.

✳ Meditation reduces DMN activity.

Creativity can as well, allowing for spontaneous processing, bypassing the Self, pulling from affective regions of the brain. The home of universal knowledge. The home of the abyss.

People living with bipolar or schizophrenia have abnormal DMNs.

Blake-like visions are hard to fit into a scanner, but I suspect much of the same.

May 2017: three months later. Second research trip. Mood and Anxiety Unit.

In six weeks, I will be there as a 100-mile tidal wave washes away my Self and I will fall

down

Charon waiting. *ABYSS*

Different building. Fifth floor. Elevator door opens and this building is tired. More of what I expected than the Youth Unit. Musky air, ornate bars that look across to a room full of green plants, slip off the edge and plunge a floor down into some unused room—chairs stacked in the corners. To the right offices. To my left, small sign:

Mood and Anxiety Unit. Everything is tired. I don't know yet how tired I am.

Cinder block walls, aged yellow, maybe once white. Low ceilings, wood brown doors. Small glass window.

Nurse doesn't look up

I'm the doctoral student here for a research project.

She gazes up, doesn't seem to know what I am talking about, but sees my badge and buzzes me in. No panopticon here, just a half door with a shelf to hand off pills and an overcrowded room of nurses. I introduce myself and place my coat and backpack on a windowsill. A nurse says he will show me around.

The layout doesn't seem to make sense, some bedrooms in a circle mixed with offices, then a broken hallway to a common area, then another circle of rooms and washrooms.

I turn into a room and meet Derek. He stands up and shakes my hand. I think he works at the hospital. But I look closer. I see his broken glasses. As we hold each other, looking into each other, I feel his gentleness and intellect. I look at him. Then longer. I feel like I know him. Or would know him, if I remember hard enough.

But then there was a sense that he was me.

It is something I don't understand yet.

He sits down and I see him drawing in a notebook. O, Derek.

✳ October 2018, I am sitting in a long room in CAMH. It is Monday and the third showing of my play *Stormshelter.* The theatre company wanted me to rename it from *Alberta #4.* Derek is sitting across from me. He has the same glasses: repaired. He dresses in a button up shirt and he looks like me. I feel like I do know him.

We watch the play. He is written in it, on the walls, on the moon, now reflecting off the scuffed tiled floor and into our minds and out of our minds. I want to share this with him. That I see him. And now he will see me.   To be witnessed.

We watch the play and I ask him if he would like to go out for a drink after. We eat chicken wings and have beers. He tells me about his band and his job. We only had eight days together a year and a half ago but he was weaved and knotted into my Being and we radiate together like brothers. Then there is a sense that he is me.

✳ Fall through the ceiling, back into the CAMH of 2017. I finish my tour and the nurse asks me if I would like to go to Tim Hortons with some of the patients and get a coffee.

Okay.

About ten of us fill into the elevator. I still don't like elevators.

As we walk out the building a twenty-year-old introduces herself to me. I meet Luanna as we slip onto the street. She says she is new. She is physically bouncing, raw human experience,

on the surface,   to the moon,   right there,

out in the open.

I smile with her as she talks at speeds that step out of time and become a nonlinear multidimensional flow of becoming. Nothing my waking mind can experience. But I have been there, will be there soon, and it's like returning home.

She asks a man on the street for a cigarette. Laughing, flirting, smiling youth and Being like a tsunami: presence. She is so charismatic she gets it. She leans close to the man and he lights the cigarette, she inhales and coughs out a chest of smoke. She laughs towards the sky,

spin,

jump,

spontaneous life unfolding, riding on an ebb and flow that these concrete buildings full of concrete minds can't sense. I look at Luanna and I start to lose myself and enter into the flow, the moment to moment, breath to breath becoming *she is*. Like some kind of priest she was waking me up. I stand on Queen Street, cool air, spring trees budding: I am ready for the sacrament.

She looks back at me.

Okay.

She is everywhere, everywhen, and everything. Yet I knew she was sick, that if she bathed in the open too long it would blister her skin and constrict her eyes, maybe beyond repair. But there was a sense of immense connection, deeper than any conventional spiritual knowing. This was untouched Knowing. Unconcealment. *Being before and within Being.* I just didn't understand that yet.

We order a coffee at Tim Hortons and sit across from each other. She talks. There is nothing for me to say, so I listen. She says she is in the middle of a manic episode. She spoke of

her new revelatory relationship with Jesus.
Happiness,   then, absolute pain
tough tough stories that are only her stories.
She was the CEO of a fashion company
                    do you want to see my designs?
Art school
She wants to be my student.
Musician, singer. In eight days, I would hear her sing. Holy voice.

Three hours earlier I land in Toronto. I couldn't say anything and she didn't need me to.

She told me about all her dreams when she gets better. She is ripe with creativity and full of hope. The netting of her mind loops to the moon and is catching the entirety of the cosmos. She is a shining light of Being. Pure becoming. The being to being *she is.* Holy Luanna.

falling
merging
opening

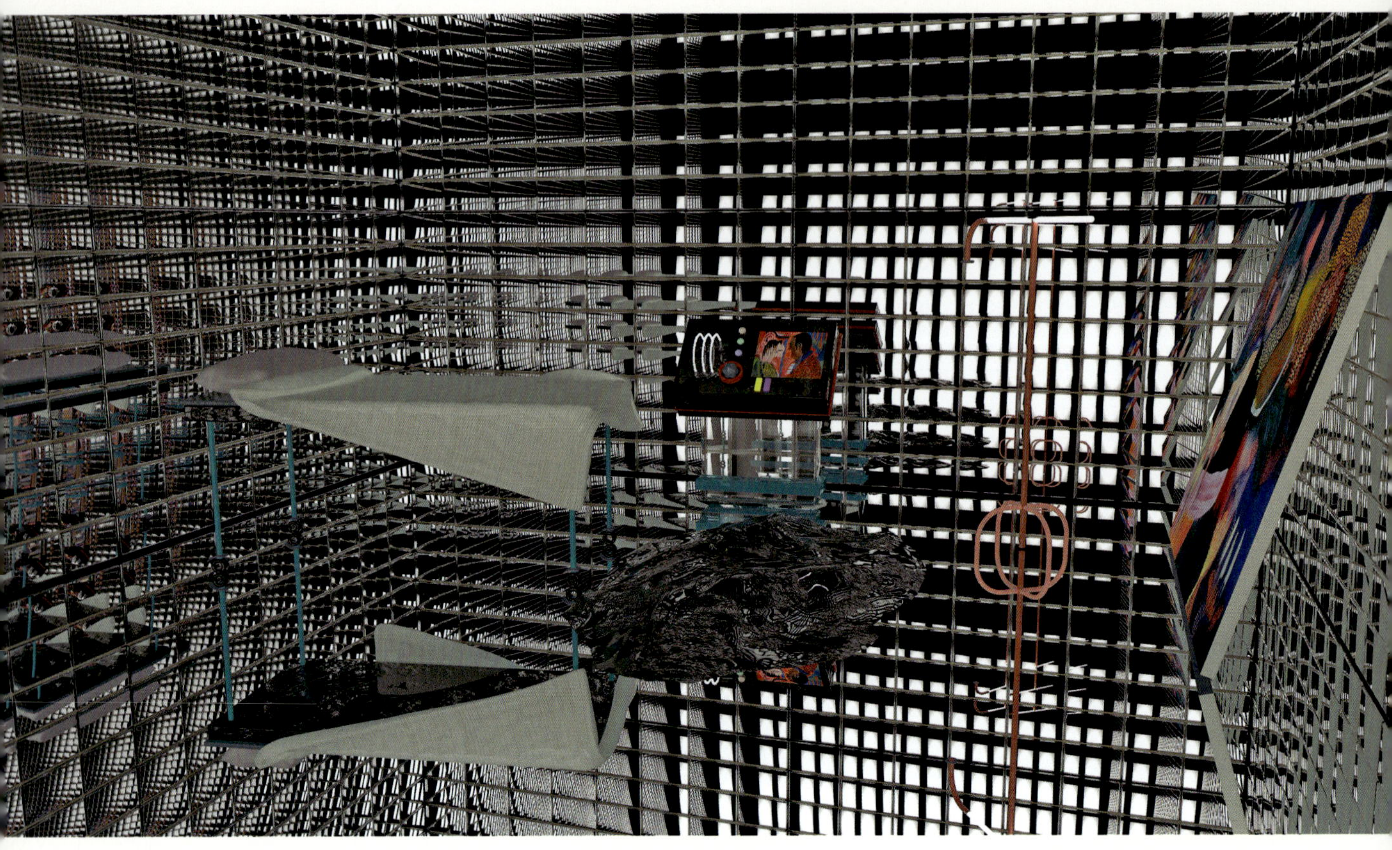

Treating Otherwise, 2018. Paintings of my psychiatrist and Luanna in a 3D-rendered environment.

There is a student from University of Toronto sitting across the table from me: depression. The depths of one's mind turned in on itself. The most concealing concealed you can be from Being. Default-Mode Network over-engaged. Self laying like a trap. I've been there.

Grey everything. Nothing,
BLACK COLOUR, NONE NUMBER. No! No! None!
no pain but ALL PAIN.
no sight, muted orange/grey like your mind can't dream anymore.
heavy eyes, vision from the void.   No one anywhere. Lone Island,
no Being comes.
Portals closed. Cosmos collapsing into the big crunch,
the   end   of   time.

I reach out to his feet and wash them, searching for a visionary angel, only to discover he *is* a visionary angel.

He looks down at me and closes his book, title: god's equation.

He is mapping god's mind, HIS mind, as it blasts and turns and radiates the mad world in *here*, out *there*, and all around. O, soul. No more hallucinating than the banker opening bank accounts or me saying I am a doctoral student studying myself.

I open my experiences to December 2018, then, September 7, 2020, now. Ginsberg emerges again, towering and breathing:

I am with you in CAMH
where you're madder than I am.
I am with you in CAMH
where you must feel very strange.
I am with you in CAMH
where you scream in a straightjacket that you're losing the sense of the actual HOME in the   a   b   y   s   s.
I'm with you in CAMH
where we wake up electrified out of the coma   by our own soul's paper wings
roaring over the moon   they've come to drop angelic VISIONS
the hospital illuminates itself
imaginary walls collapse
O Milky Way, run outside
O Canada, shock of mercy
the eternal fall is here
O victory forget ~~You~~,we are free!

I'm with you in CAMH

in my dreams you walk dripping from a cosmic-journey on the rivers across Canada in tears to the door of my mind in this heavenly night.

I'm with you in CAMH

where fifty more shocks will never return your soul to its body again from its pilgrimage to a cross into the abyss...

You ask me, but I can't attend your electroconvulsive therapy sessions. I think they will let me but I can't let myself. Sorry frightened soul. Drifting in the boat of the Self, nowhere near land, no guiding stars, lost moon, forever night.

At lunch you come back into the room in a wheelchair, head to the side, no more anything behind your eyes. Shocked out Being and left as electrified flesh with a face I still know.

I see you into infinity, friend. Radiant jewel, scuffed and no-one. As I look past your eyes into the void, I see a room.

I don't know what to do. So I do what the patients are doing. I am so tired,
tired,
maybe some part of me wants to be admitted.

Derek, Luanna, and I continue to fuse and express together, one. It would have been easy to fall with them, but I need to stay attentive, open.

Head up, look around the room.

Depressed patients are harder to connect with. The most we can share are the TV commercials selling us solvents. Many have tremors and hollowed faces as they detox. But I watch TV with them, we talk a bit, Default-Mode Network laying like a trap, turned in on themselves, lonely islands, but they are on their journey and I am on mine.

I look across the room to a table in the corner and walk over. This small woman looks up to me, terrified by my introduction. I ask to sit and, trembling, she invites me to commune. She only looks forward into a mirror across the room, never into me and we begin to talk about
ghosts,
flying out this fifth-floor window through Toronto skies,
and visions.
Luanna sits close and listens.

Hero dreams, vibrant scented visions, sweeping storms, solar flares, and quasars. She tells me madness stories from another plane. I have no idea what I am doing here, sitting across from a frightened soul, wailing before Being, burning with Being, unravelling her telomeres before Being, scratching her arm, scratching herself to the bone, scratching to find the marrow and imprinting drawings of ~~You~~ or ~~Me~~,
or crumpled desires
as she weeps and I weep
below the roiling deck of the Self.

She trembles when she speaks.
I look at the whites of her eyes and I don't
recognize the reflections shining back at me
(stardust falling off a comet),

but her withholding gaze pierces me, forcing me to project into places I can't go alone, eliciting sensations,

the sensations of sensations,
as I look at the psychiatric room, aged white cinderblock walls, saddened windows, hollow locks, yellow sun, forever exploding pure becoming, filling my eyes with its illumination, imagining a few billion years away when it will grow large, filling the sky, becoming an infinite plane between the horizon and light, consuming Mercury, then Venus, then me. I lift back up into Mind, reach out, World sheltering, blinking for two jewels on Indra's Net reflecting, yet
no Earth between her and I to negotiate, collapse, void—
and when I look into her eyes I see an expanse I did not yet know.—void,
and

I am afraid,
then,
she begins repeating mantras to herself,
shaman,
under her breath,
shaman
forgetting this room,
her,
me,
shaman,
summoning force,
repeating and
repeating,
shaman
circling,
gaining and gaining,
down and down
shaman and doom,
then,
she becomes a column of air, I can see right through her to the wall, a visible Charon,
then,
she is rising up the abyss with sheer mystical presence, within me and around the room.
then,
She looks down and down in me and speaks,
repeating herself,
then,
terrifying me,
again,
reciting numinous sounds of no-sense,
held in suspense
as our souls collapse
into each other,
then,

she shoves the table away from her
a mountain rises, reaching to god,
she erodes the sun; black
and stands tall before me and starts screaming.
Full of force, shaman, shaman, shaman, filling each
inhale, evaporating everything on the out breath,
she is summoning something I have never
seen before.
I fall back and take in the sermon. Holy!
Screaming Holy! Bracing! Bare! Naked! Skin is holy! Her breathing is holy!
I am holy!
Luanna starts arguing with her that she is
terrifying people,
but I remain silent. Shaman, I was transfixed in this being
unfolding and
expressing
before me, before Being.
Becoming.

Hallucinations summoning fear, bliss, we triumph, fallen power,
breath to breath,
death,
resurrection, illumination,
death,
resurrection, illumination,
death,
resurrection, illumination,
madness, fire
resurrection, dreaming,
incarnation, hallucination,
suffering, compassion
awakening
merging
no-one
Being
one,
collapse, infinite collapse,
finite breath, glimpsing,
blistering, event horizon,
charged and rotating,
terror,
delight, desire,
ascension, home

The nurses rush in but stop at the door.
Everyone is transfixed, submitting to the sermon.
She has become life and death hanging in the room,
    doom.

She awakens me, terrified, into the dream. I feel my sins weeping, suffering,
my last breath, falling out at once, cascading down to the floor, rampaging
down the halls, out onto the streets of Toronto, of Canada, O sorrowful soul
I don't want

She glides to the mirror on the wall. She looks at herself, repeating holy
words from some other
        World
she starts touching her face
bodysuit
someone else
peering through the window of eyes
hollow face evaporating before pure
Being
repeating archetypal words from all
life on this planet to her, connecting her
to the beginning of time, each word
imprinted with the Cosmic Microwave
Background,
and the ever evaporating star she is
forge out of
climbing up and up into her soul
a spirit thrust into a body to have
HUMAN experiences
but she falls to the floor with me over her
shoulder
she bends down further and looks into
the whirlpool at her feet
face reflecting and distorting, ripping,
falling, and disappearance.
it goes still, mirror ocean, like a Blake
poem never written,
then,
SCREAMING,
horror, death, destruction, resurrection,
and death again
, raging, pain,
And,

she is hit by a gamma-ray burst from a
far off galaxy.
She collapses to the ground with gravity.

The sermon is over, the nurses leave their post along the wall and grab her under her arms.

Her feet drag along the floor, hospital gown falling off her naked crumpled body, and she is screaming about the being in the mirror, the mirror that holds onto no-thing.

I fall to the ground, slip through the floor, floor after floor, soil, clay, granite, magma, iron,
origin.

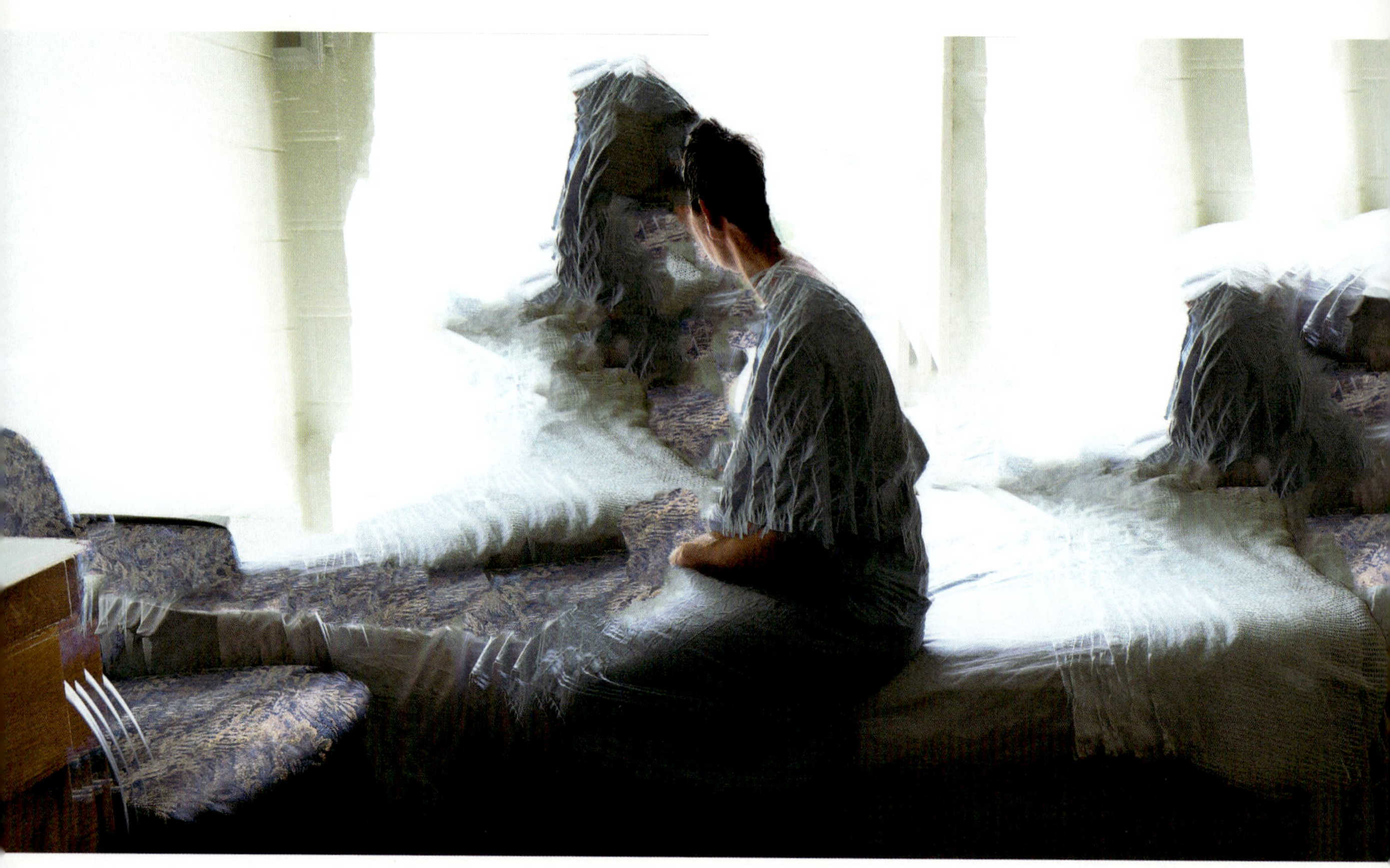

Derek staring into the portal, the thin place between waking and dreaming, sanity and madness.

May 2017: Derek, Luanna, and I continue to connect. Planning artworks, going to the gym and playing sports, going to therapy sessions, long walks through Trinity Bellwoods Park, Luanna jumping and signing, Derek in a long coat, and looking at the stonewall along the hospital built by patients in the 1800s. *Their labour, frustrations, and time.*

One day Derek and I go with a volunteer and sign up for a meditation session. I have never meditated and don't expect anything other than to be bored. But I sit, cross my legs, close my eyes, and listen to the volunteer's voice. My mind runs, slipping from thought to thought, mental string to mental string. But her voice has some kind of presence and I listen.

The mental space behind my eyes begins to expand. I continue to sit and listen. Her voice becomes distant, like there is more space, all-space, some kind of force driving the expansion of the space behind my eyes, my consciousness. I feel some kind of dissent, down and down. Warmer and warmer, shelter. I didn't yet know about spaciousness. I am floating.

Then, a gentle gesture that the session is over, but I'm not in the room. I try to open my eyes and as I do I feel some kind of ascension. Slipping back into the dream. Worlding this world. My mind feels tingly and clear. Very clear. I look at Derek and we are looking into each other for the first time.

✳ I still couldn't get ethics approval to do next to anything in the hospital, but they let me come in and observe. I did get approval later but never made it back to the hospital, my madness was becoming too frequent. A few days into my stay at the Mood and Anxiety Unit, the unit manager let me bring in a camera, as long as the patients weren't identifiable.

As soon as the camera comes in Derek and Luanna burst with ideas. None of which we could do, but we slipped into the flow. Derek wants a video of him in a hospital gown walking into his room. I record it and follow him in as he sits on his bed. Later, I stack all the stills together and make this image of him—gazing into the abyssal portal of madness. An invitation to look.

Next, I follow Luanna around the halls and she wants me to take photos of her. I listen to her but I knew I couldn't use any of these. Just the flow of breath to breath with them.

She sits in window sills gazing over Toronto, dances, flows like water down the hallways lined with rooms holding minds, reaches to the ceiling pressing down with antipsychotics dishonouring the becoming she is. She lays in her bed laughing and talking at speeds describing every artwork we would never make across this lifetime we have fallen into. She contains multitudes.

Derek goes into his drawer and pulls out all these notebooks his mom had brought him: he wants to show them to me. He hands me a couple CDs of his band. I look through his notebook: worn, warm, lyrics bursting at every seam, madness. He takes out a piece of paper and starts drawing and writing on it, of all the art we want to make together. Years later, I find that note tucked in one of my notebooks. I feel to Derek's gentleness and intellect. I look closer. I can barely tell the difference between his notes and mine.

Luanna, Derek, and I are sitting in his room, looking at his notebooks, and dreaming. Derek says he wants to tear apart his room to show the chaos in his mind.

(later a nurse tells me he did just that when he was first admitted, before the meds had slowed him down.)

He destroys his room and I photograph it.

Then Luanna wanted her room to be documented. So I set up the camera and we set the composition together. She doesn't do anything to her room.

Over the next few days, we document a bunch of patients' rooms. We sit in the common area watching TV and commercials, editing photos on my laptop, everyone on the unit joining in.

We talk about mad things. God, Illumination, medications, electric shocks, UFOs, ghosts, secret military, pilgrimages we will never make to each other across the unimaginable space between Edmonton and Toronto. Bus rides in the night, holy communions, blinking, blinded, headlights that crash us into our bodies and remind us of the dream.

I never felt more at home than I did with you two. No walls, no sadness, no pain, just recovery. Your recovery and my recovery. Haunted by Being, bathing in Being, blistered by Being, constricted, falling, merging together in the night time, staring over a Toronto sky-scape, condos, Queen Street, Trinity Bellwoods Park, where the three of us walk under trees budding for the spring, bringing new life, spontaneous, expressing, flowing, breathing the air we share between our conversations, that falls around our mouths, finding homes in each of our minds.

Now my memories are fading. Luanna, do I really remember what you look like? Words slipping out of form, left with sensations. So I close my eyes, and sense these sensations coursing, collecting across time, stillness, then raging white rapids that fall out of the mountain of skull and down, down, down into the music room...eternal place in my Mind.

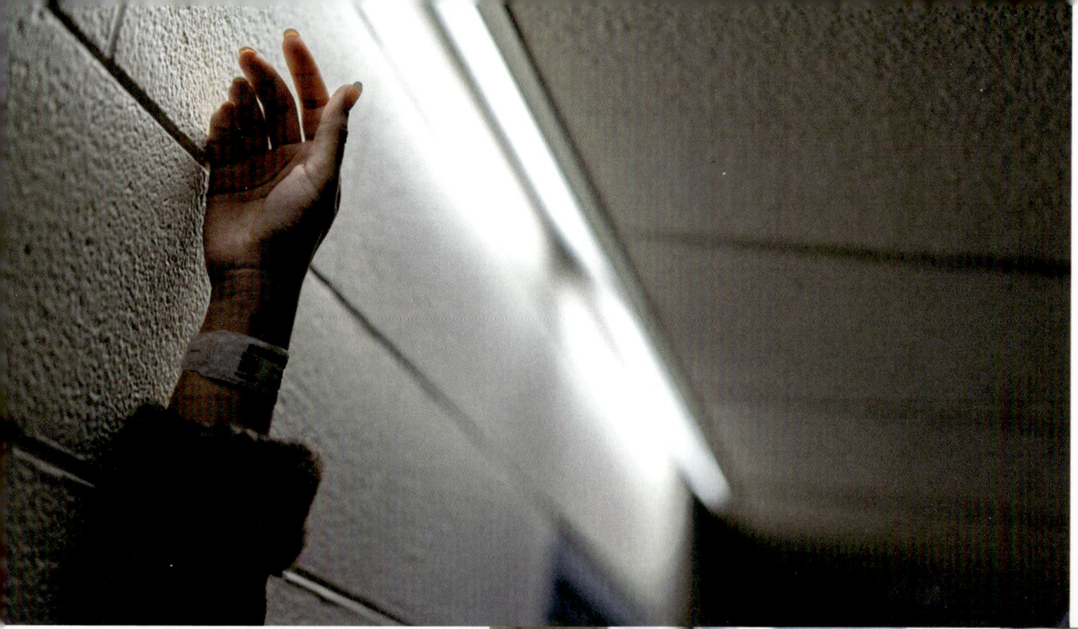

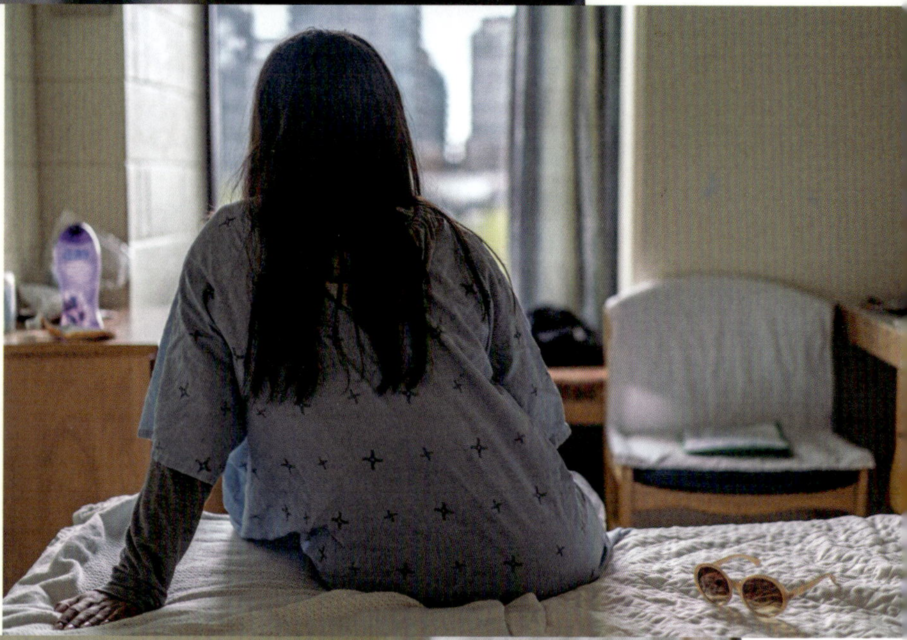

(Top) Around CAMH with Luanna. (Middle) Luanna and sunglasses. (Bottom) Luanna posing in her bed.

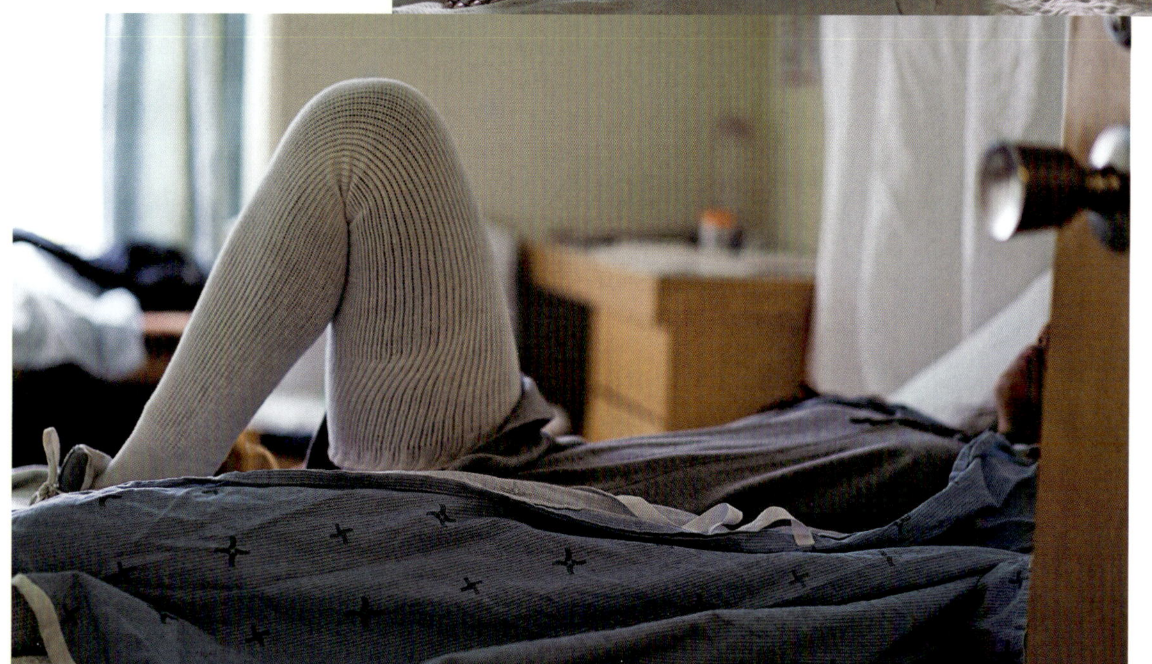

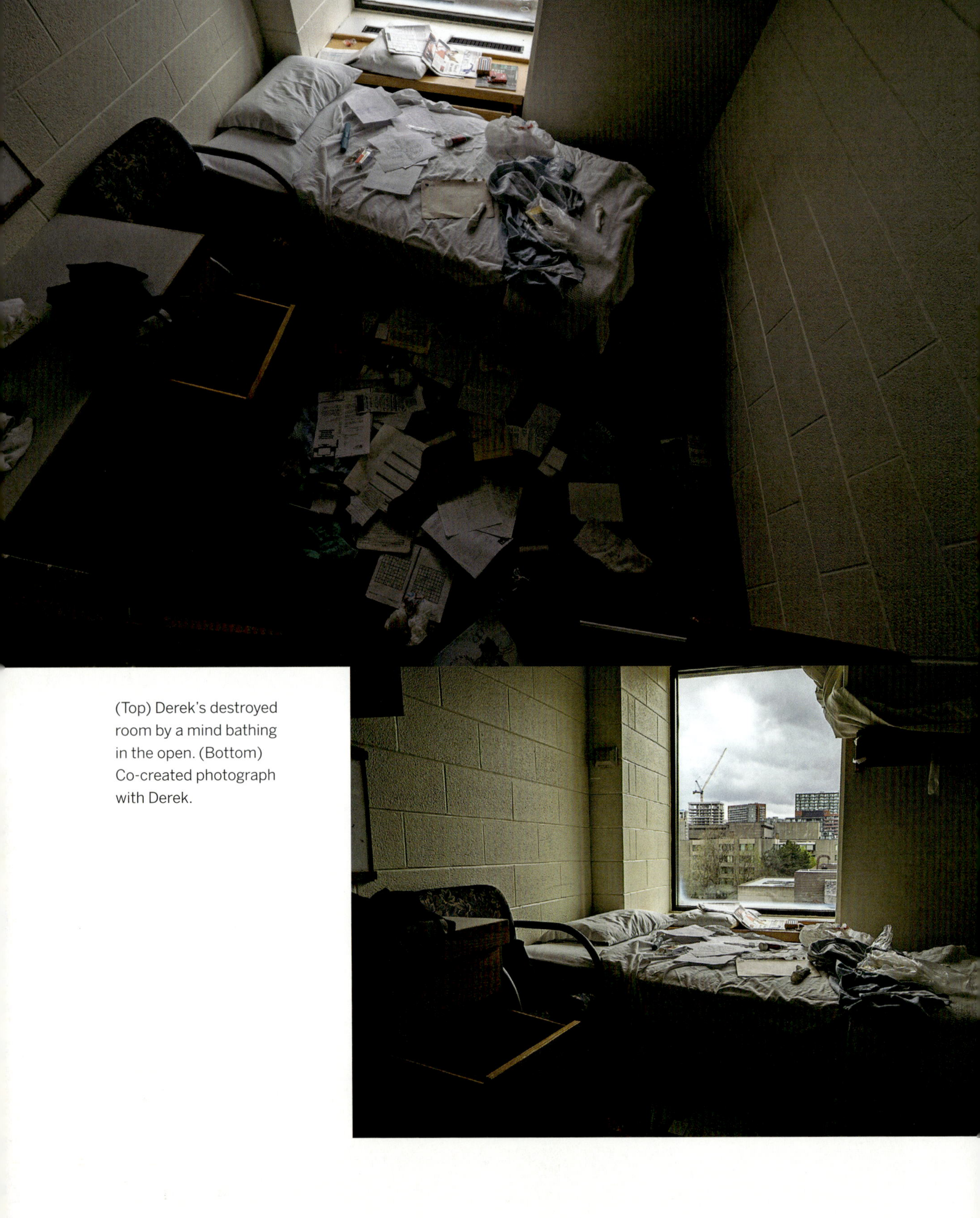

(Top) Derek's destroyed room by a mind bathing in the open. (Bottom) Co-created photograph with Derek.

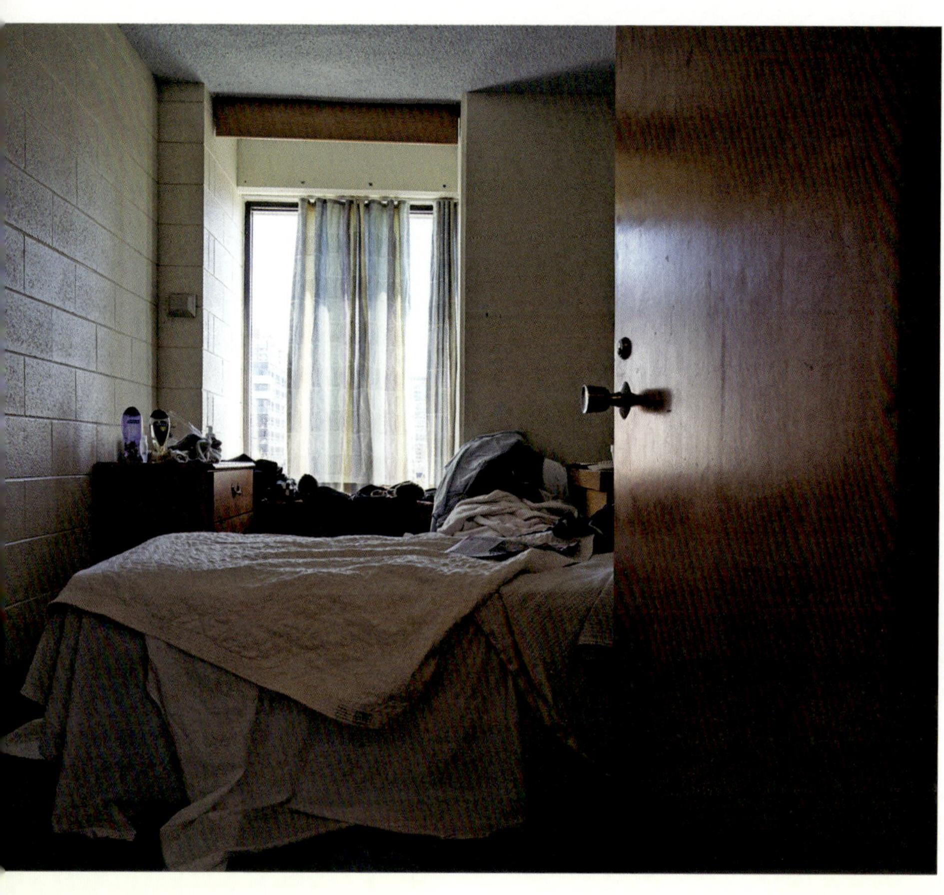

(Top) Luanna's room left just as is. (Bottom) *Creating Otherwise*, 2018. Derek's room,,,and mine.

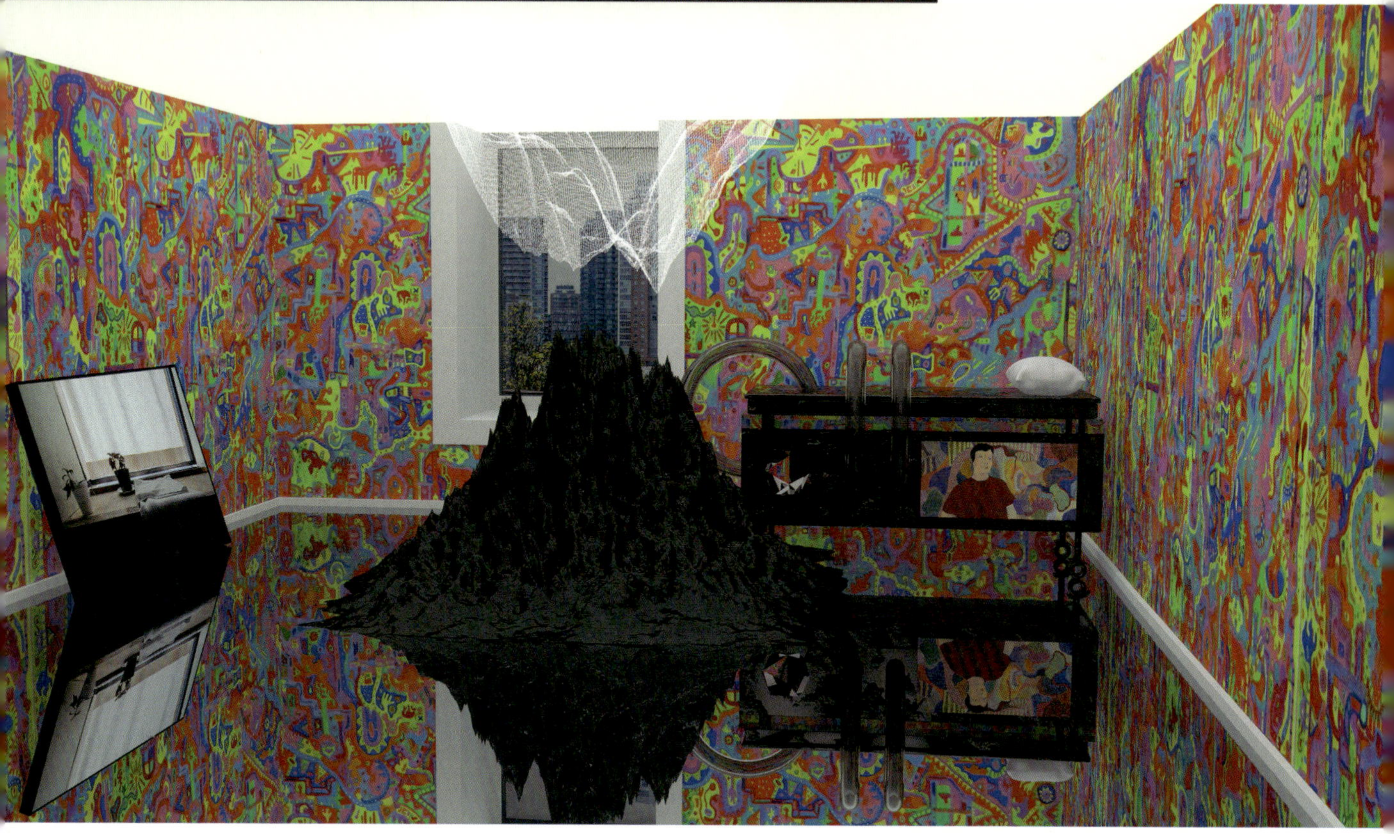

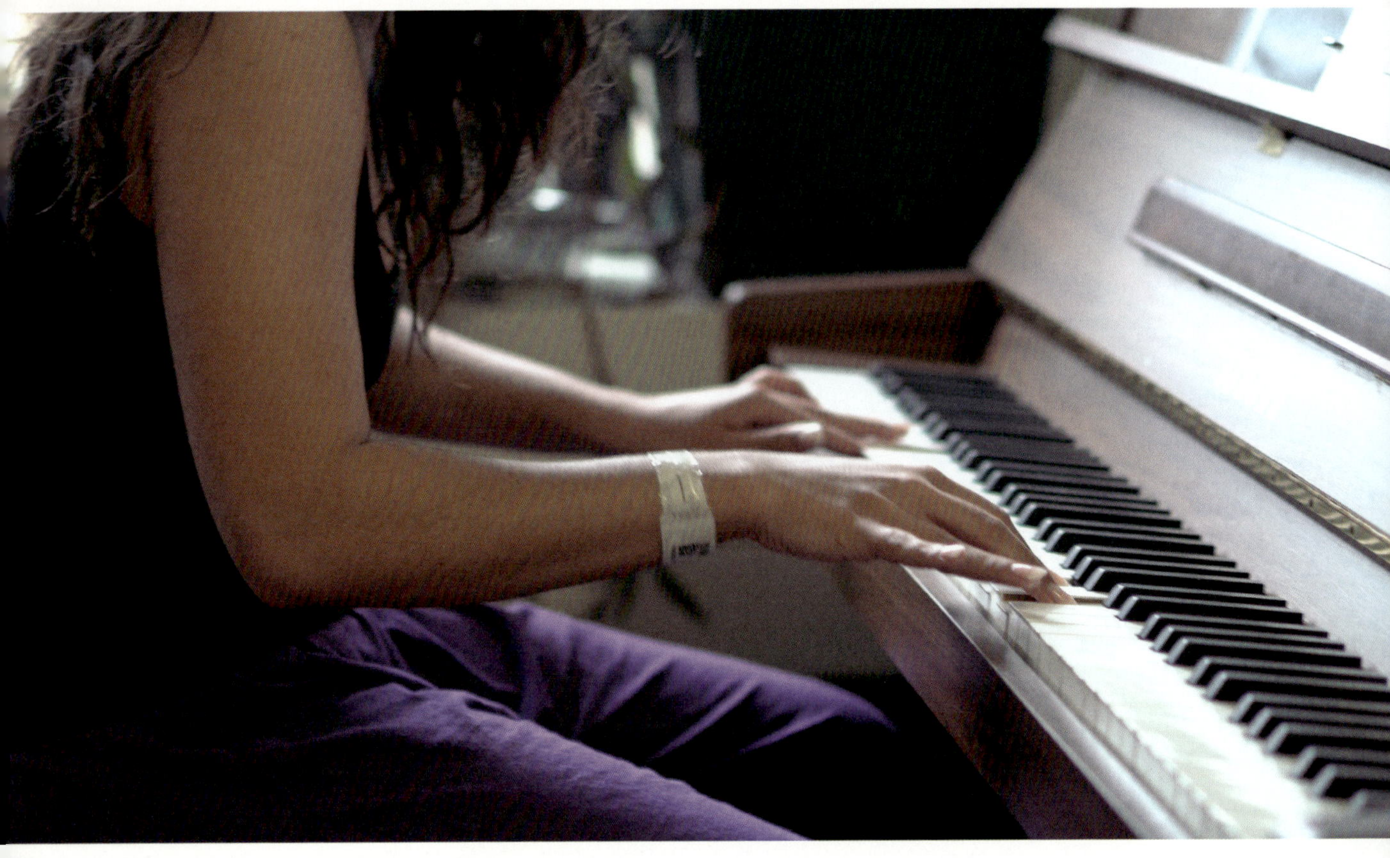

Luanna imposing on the piano.

We share a madness experience, coarse and twisted, knotted, strung along a stretching expanse. My last day felt like the LAST DAY. I will hug Derek. I will hug Luanna.

Before: we find our way into the music room. Outside the locked doors, down the hall. Over my shoulder, gazing and slipping through the hall and I wonder if I can just walk out, or if I am a patient. Time rotating, everything all at once, maybe I would be in that hall forever. Six weeks later, in Mind, I would be, we were just slightly out of alignment. Again, writing these words September 12, 2020, Being shifting, slipping, the circle game.

Derek borrows a guitar from the hospital and plays us music and sings. Luanna sits at the piano in the room and finds her way through some chords. Slowly,

press press change press

Heaven

A few days before I hear her on the phone crying with her dad. He doesn't understand what she was going through, wounded by everything that came before. Over the past eight days, Luanna has changed. Before: so confident she would return to her life, the place of all the tough things that led her here, in this room, singing outside of Mind. But now she was coming down, coming to realize all the things she had been through and where she now wanted to go. I record her hands as she improvises on the piano, singing a hymn,

—I am losing control,

over and over, like a mantra, breath to breath, a meditation on Being.

I collapse with her voice, O god I wish I could share her voice.

She slips eyes close, hands move, stumble,

but always finding the chord.

I am losing control with her, moment to moment. Derek looks like a priest presiding over a sermon,

some kind of revelation was unfolding, and we were the lone witnesses.

O, Luanna, crying a cry of layers, a cry of recognition, screaming a mantra that shatters the imaginary wall of this imaginary hospital,

no more cinder blocks, locks, windows looking at expensive condos for people hallucinating sanity.

Connection. Deeper than an embodied awareness, more like a geological awareness,

long and vast, and
much closer to the ground that I ever thought I
could be, now
floating in the air of Toronto,   some Canada,   all three of us   t
here,
no-one, one,
ecstatic glimpses of Being, yes.

When I went manic I thought of you two often.
What would that illness journey looked
like if we could have been together. Are
you well? I'm sitting beside an ocean my
feet are cooling in.   British
Columbia.
Trying to remember something. ///
Ginsberg, again \\\

I see the best minds of my generation ILLUMINATED by madness, falling,
dissolving and no-one.
Dragging themselves through Canada's mental sky at dawn, looking for
connection, anything.
Angel-minded maniacs burning for the ancient heavenly connection to the
starry eyes in the hallucination that there ever is a night.

Strange, now, to think of you,
gone without hospital bracelets or
VISIONS,
while I hike on the rolling
mountains of British Columbia.
HOLY!
Dreaming back through life, ~~Your~~ time—
and ~~mine~~ accelerating towards
the event horizon, the final
moment
where all directions are
down,
the flowers burning south,,, in California,
clogging my sky, itching my
lungs—and scared of what is to
come after,
looking back on the Mind, in the Mind itself
that saw a Canadian dream
a flash away, the great

dream of Me, or You
and phantom hope, or a crumpled
abyss that always existed.
Waiting.
—like a poem in the dark—escaped back to
Oblivion—
No more to say, and nothing to weep for
but the Being of Beings in the
Dream! trapped in disappearance,
sighing, screaming!   Buying and
selling hallucinations, worshipping
THE Dream.
Derek, Luanna, awakened, rambling as
they lept off from the riverbank,
washing in time and slipping down
and down,

whirlpool, untouched,
no breath needed, simply,

plainly,

Being.

I

2017: I get back from CAMH on a May Sunday. I wake up the next morning, drive to the UofA, and start teaching a spring class that will run for the next three weeks. Everything was easy, slipping into place, but I was slipping, in an unknown way, like my orbit was shifting, gravity waves pushing at me, tectonic plates locking.

On the last day of class, I present at the Department of Psychiatry's research day. I get up, show a single slide, read a statement about cancer, and never look at the crowd. I walk out the room and Andy follows me out. He asks how my family is doing. He looks further into me, he asks me how I am doing. I feel the tears behind the dam and say I need a new psychiatrist. Something isn't right. He says he will help me find a new one.

A few days later, I am in Calgary attending a meeting with some of the top mental health researchers in Alberta. I am there to learn, so I listen. When we finish, I get into my car and drive out to the Rocky Mountains: Banff National Park. I look up at Cascade Mountain and see a billion years of time like glyphs of geological awareness. Snow-capped, summer air, clouds hanging, rain pouring, me pouring a bottle of bourbon as I slip into my hotel bed. Tired eyes and a misting mind.

The next morning Maria meets me in Banff. We walk down from the Banff Centre for the Arts and find a rock overhanging a stream. She looks into me and says I can't continue at this pace. That I won't make my best work if this is my Being, so concealed, twisted in on itself.

I look up at the canopy, sun casting light and shadow on Tunnel Mountain like an Ansel Adams photograph. Everything around me wants to push up and up. But I don't listen to Maria.

I get home and have ideas for physically constructing psychiatric rooms and photographing them. The times weren't synced yet and I would have to wait a year to begin the *Otherwise* series. Early June, when I walk in the house Candace walks out and flies to the Maritimes to present at a conference. My mom and I take care of the girls, Mary one, but she is teething and has me up for hours each night. Sleep is one of my biggest defenses against shifting moods, right up there with meds. But all the tectonic plates had been collecting and pressing over the months

and

slip   a seismic wave that evaporates the imaginary Self, tsunami of pure Being. Radiating in the top of my skull and out the top of my skull,

goodbye, Default-Mode Network

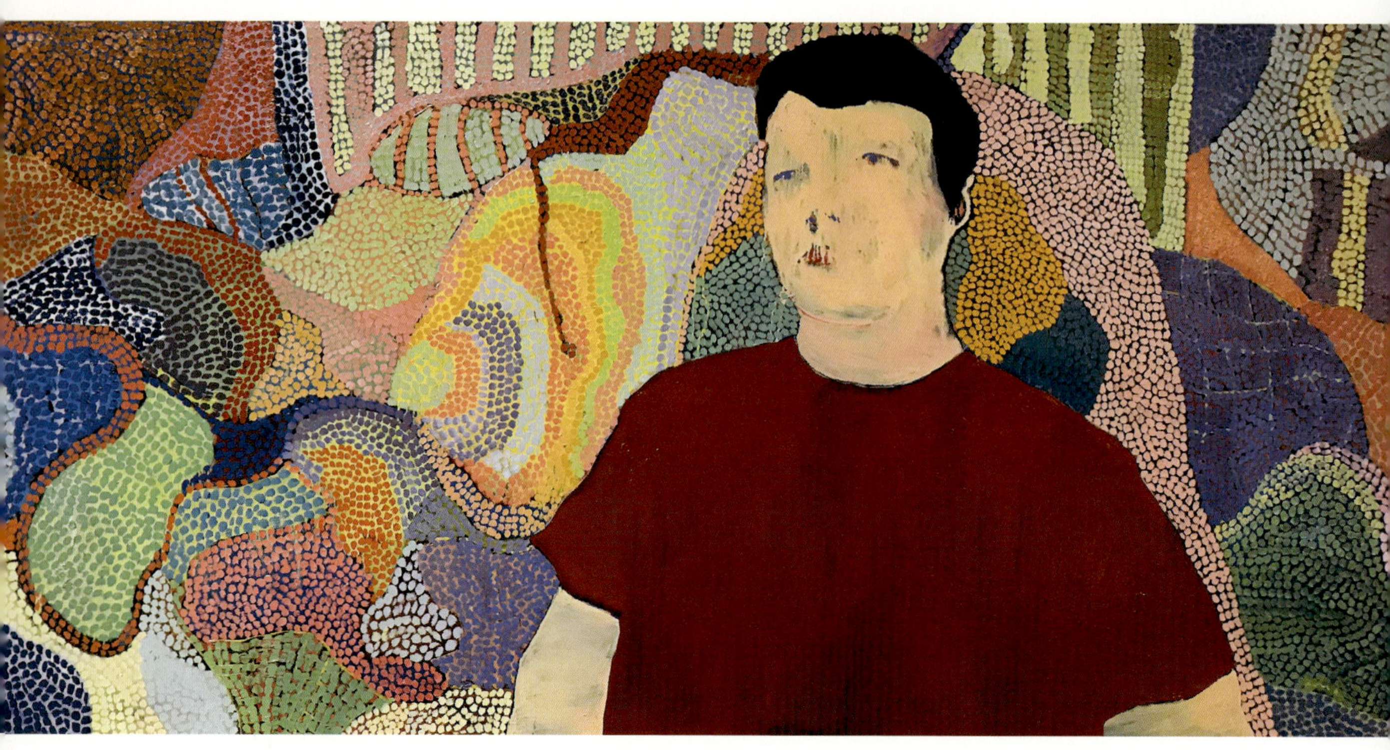

June 18: Mania.

goodbye Self, goodbye happiness, security, so long, June 2017, then July
goodbye home, family
No psychiatrist. No pills. Cobbling together old meds, imagining what a doctor would say, in the end, nowhere near enough.
And so I went d
o
w
n

II

The first week is disappearance. Perfect mirror, holding onto nothing,
no memories
stick.
Bourbon to slow my mind, trying to fall asleep, fall back in the
dream,

ALL COLOUR, INFINITY particles, eroding
hallucination,
every grain of sand
eons all at once,
everywhen
pushing my hand
through mountains
finding all the SPACE
between everything.
Quantum field
Indra's Net, jewel,
and all of everything
blasting my Being.
Connected beyond
humanity,
beyond life,
beyond
Earth,
off in the
cosmos
the birth
of a new
universe.

A runaway nuclear reaction,   neutrons scattering,   splitting the atoms of
the imaginary Self,
    gone
        gone, empty, emptied,
                emptiness
Mania, the great teacher, with awe and terror,   forget
        past,   future   illusions, mental
        algorithms,
        no, now is Illumination   radiation   gamma-ray burst
        No-where to hide, no-sense in saying okay, no-say in anything,
        plainly, simply, becoming
                    absolute flow.
                    out in the open ocean.

Then, brown canvas,   made years ago in art school.
Ancient paints: expression.
I see you, Derek,   then spray you with turpentine, I can't see your face right now,
hiding from gamma-ray bursts.

Pink dots flowing out the back of your head,   muted green striped with
                    yellow are your window's bars.
Full of Being, I create the right side, but as I spill down the left,   pain, disbelief,
                    my kid's in pain, O Candace!
        the left's colours harmonize less, something is slipping down and
        down in me.
    New depths, completely uncharted,   open ocean, empty night sky,
                other than obliteration
                oblivion
                home
dot after dot: meditation. One thread tether hanging onto body,   alive maybe
                        dead.
Each day spills into the next, painting pouring out of mind.
Madness,   gone,   my family goes through the unimaginable.

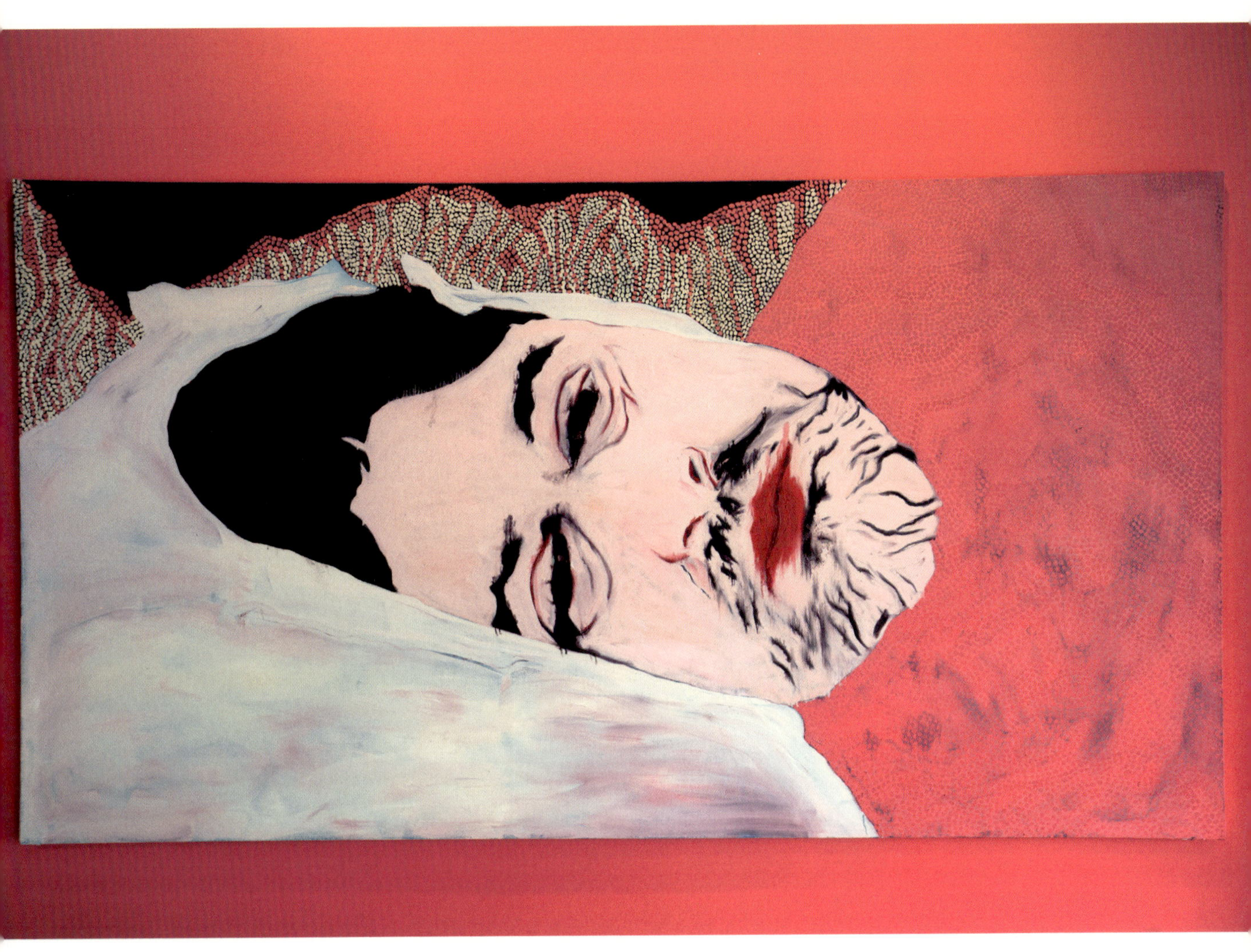

June 22: from
Father's Day.

III

June 18, 2017: Father's Day.

The day I can't remember the faces of my children. I feel terrible for what I said.

When I wake up with Candace by me we talk.

Then she leaves and I lift my phone.

A wasted reflection covering my wasted mind.

I wish I could be with Derek and Luanna.

I take a photograph as I lay on my side, death hung in the room.

My eyelids feel stiff and dry from the salt in evaporated tears and my mind is a fog from the antipsychotics pressing on my Being like an asteroid.

I build a 6 × 10 foot stretcher and paint myself.

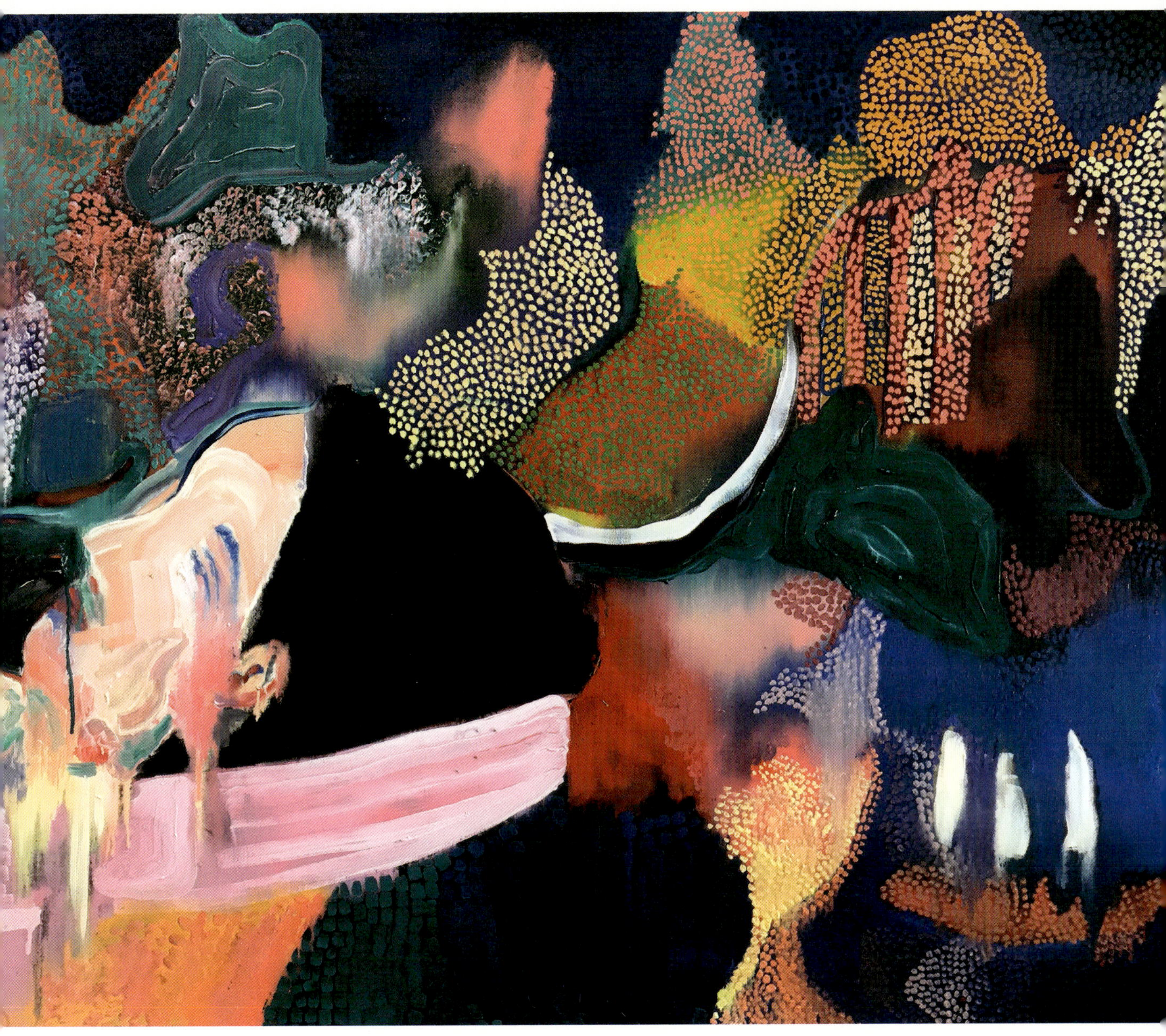

June 23: Luanna.

IV

June 23:

I see you Luanna, like mental jewels in
northern Ontario
a Canadian landscape
pale pink boat on
Lake Nipissing
three lanterns illuminating
the starless night
you lay in the bath, searching for shelter, melting before
the supermassive blackhole's Hawking radiation,

k

T

=

ħ

g

2

π

c

=

ħ

c

4

ϖ

r

s

hammering spiritual storm, tearing through the fabric of spacetime,

c =

R

S

,

2

G

M

then

G

ab

:

=

R

ab

–

1

2

R

g

ab

=

κ 0 T

ab +Λ

...
evaporating incarnation
toil and blood ,
vibrant spectrum is the VISION. road
grown - over
I'm
out in t he wilder ness ,
Being, now void
of form
column of air , turb u le nce,
aching pain | love
the webbing of the M ind grabbing
neutron stars , bl asting qu asars,
pulling t he moon to the Earth
under my covers ,
Sun on close approach filling
the sky
home evaporates t he ground
extends
everywhere
Sun filling t h e sky
ground stretching to t h e edge of the
observable universe, 90
billion ligh t - years
Sun expanding , dark energy creating
allspace, I stand , the lone witness of the
end *of* *the* *u* *niverse*
t he sun becomes an infinite plane
above the Earth becomes an infinite ground
I a m between two infinite planes
and , slip , lights out,
forever night
I look to t he halo of light to
my left
I look at you , Luanna . ~~You~~
say
come in, hold on,

breathe in

breathe out

some kind of mental shelter,   dilating, falling, *a being with and within Being.*
Becoming.

I was burned out from exhaustion,
buried below the event horizon,

poisoned,
ruptured,
hunted,
ravaged,
come,   she
said

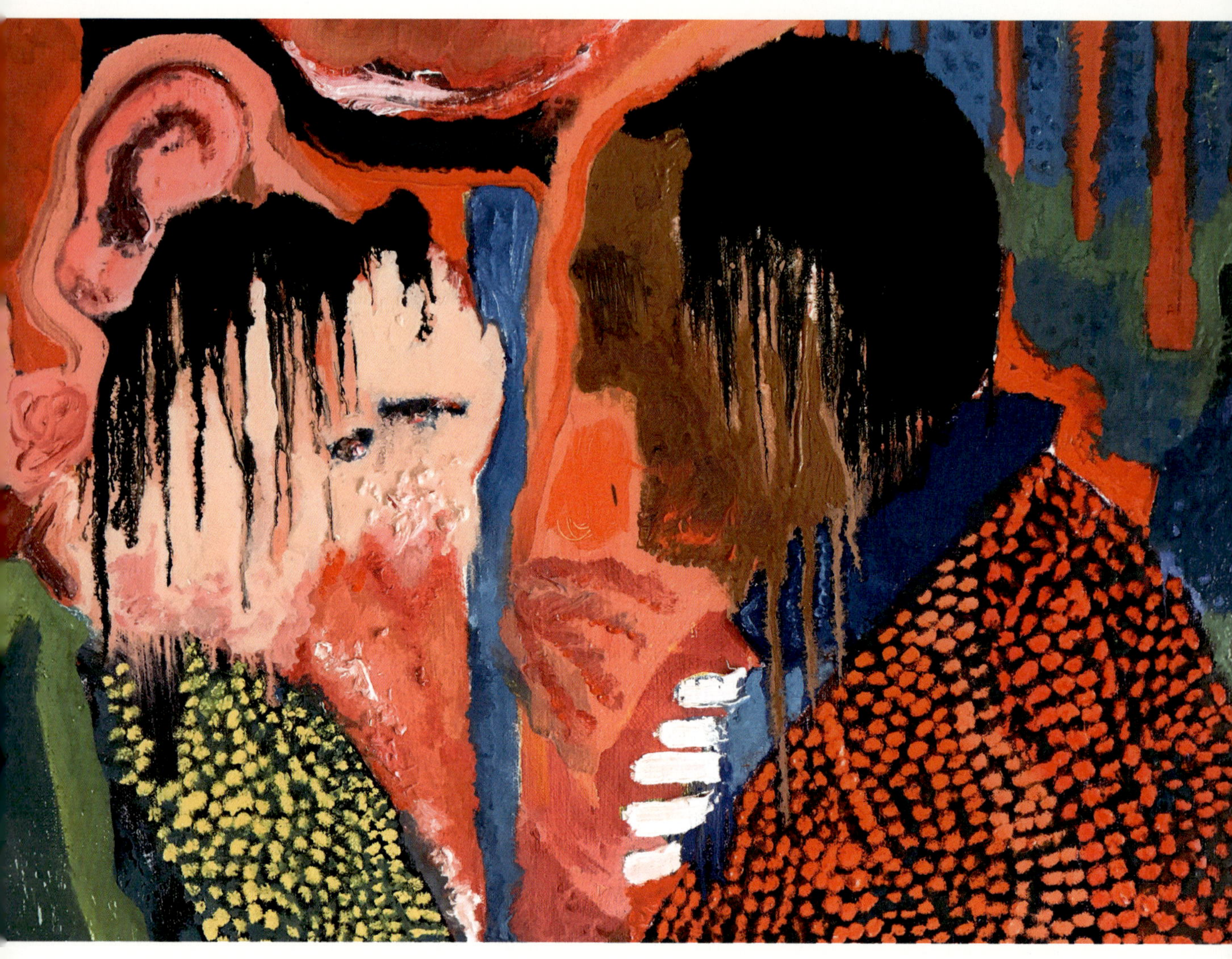

June 25: Psychiatrist.

V

June 25: Today is the most pain I have ever experienced.
I see my old psychiatrist,   the one that did all these tough things to me.
Treated me like electrified flesh.
Once I bring Elliot to my appointment and he talks to her kindly.
He talks to me about routines, lifestyle,   the things I would
find are
the actual cure in
years to come.
But the pills, the withdrawal, the meds to balance the meds to balance the meds, once on Parkinson's meds, shaking
so twisted in on myself that I couldn't breathe. I don't know why he did that to me,

I'm talking to him outside Mind.   I think I am about to die.
I can't fall asleep and painted and painted, feeling like the mental space between my ears and behind my eyes was collapsing into a charged black hole and this was an event horizon that I couldn't come back from.
I was dissolving with solvents in every way possible, spewing nothingness on his blind eyes and disintegrating ears.
In this moment, I doubt psychiatry like I doubt my existence.
In this moment, I don't believe I exist.
Before me a mirror forms and I gaze into it: transfixed
it is like a sermon
~~i~~ don't recognize the being in
the mirror
the beings in the mirror
they scream at me
the mirror that holds no-thing

(Top) June 26: For him.
(Bottom) June 27:
For Jesse.

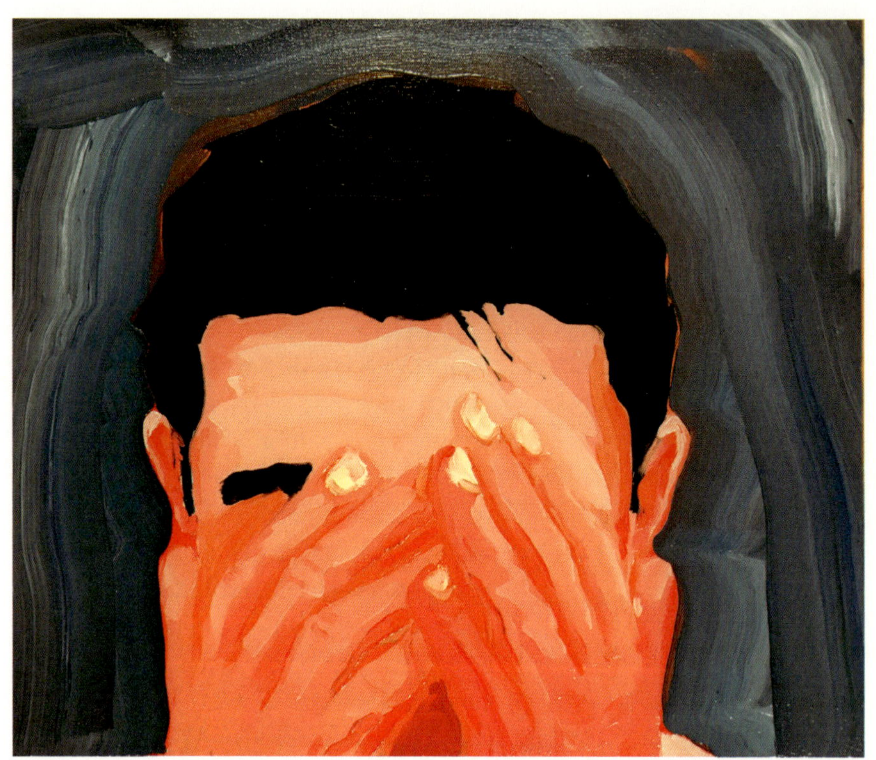

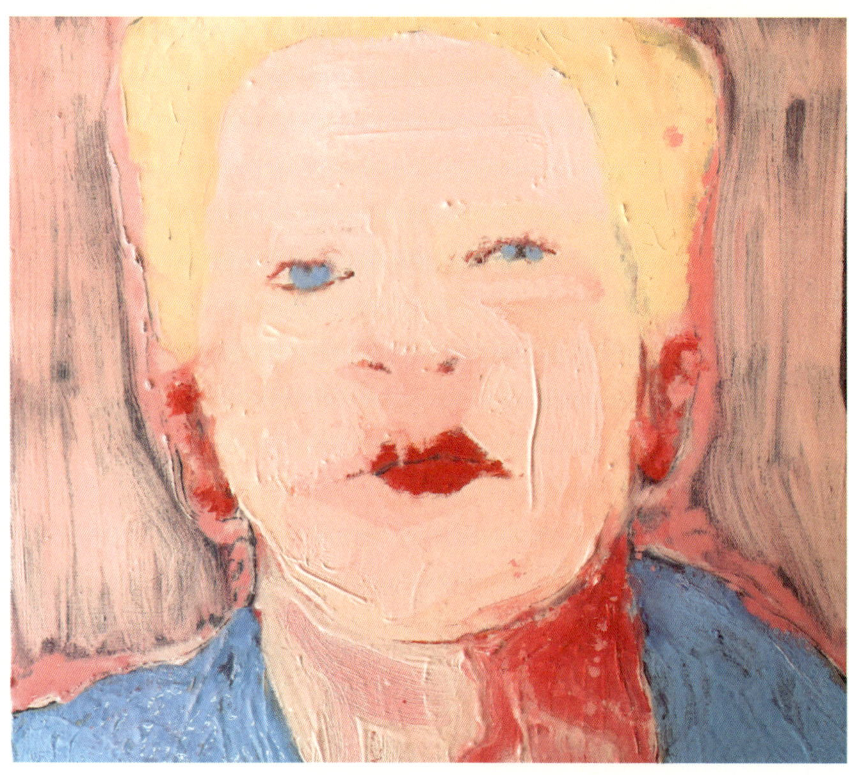

VI

By June 28, I start seeing my new psychiatrist. She gave me a high dose of antipsychotics. It wasn't comforting, but horrifying. They were sealing off Being, the Being that was blasting me like a gamma-ray burst from another galaxy. The kind that was showing me everything

the birth of the world
my birth or death
me, plain as day, no comforting haze
filling my consciousness with primordial images

then, it gave me a kiss. A kiss Candace and I just have as my feet get weighted with lead and I came to spend time with her. Reconciling the unimaginable.

June 25 is the last stand of my mania, clawing for breath, screaming, Psychiatrist!

Holding onto the Kingdom of Illumination, the pure space of the open, with Being, outside Time.

June 26: the kids are in bed and I make a painting with my head in my hands. No disintegration, no solvents, just some paint and colour. On June 27, I construct a 6 x 9 canvas, taking most of the day. No simple affair on a hot day, listening to Johnny Cash's *American Recordings* blasting out the garage door, exposing my mind to the neighbourhood. And then painting a small portrait of Jesse from CAMH. I take my pills and try to sleep.

June 28: morning, a bit less confusing, pain. I have a nuclear furnace of energy. But the energy wasn't blinding me, but one that had the right lenses and mirrors to focus it through my body and mind and onto the canvas. I painted the ear, sprayed some solvent and a muted green dripped, but this wasn't about disintegrating anymore. So I moved onto the hand and filled each stroke with mountains of paint. Carving out a knuckle, a bone, some flesh.

Everything slowed after that. I write field notes as I continue to come down from heaven. In November, I would include them in *Alberta #3.*

I hug Ellie Mary radiating Candace
I look to my mom, we are going through *it* again.
I look to my dad, holding me in the garage, crying, crying
a generational cry. I see generations of my ancestors
holding their children. I look to the blue sky out the garage
door and just then all of my ancestors look at it too.
I see myself holding Ellie. Mary. myself as a child.
I fall into Candace, the love of my life, everywhere and
everywhen at the centre of my universe. I fall because
falling is easier than resisting. And so we fall.
We share a lifetime together, coarse and twisted, knotted,
strung along a stretch expanse of Being and Time.

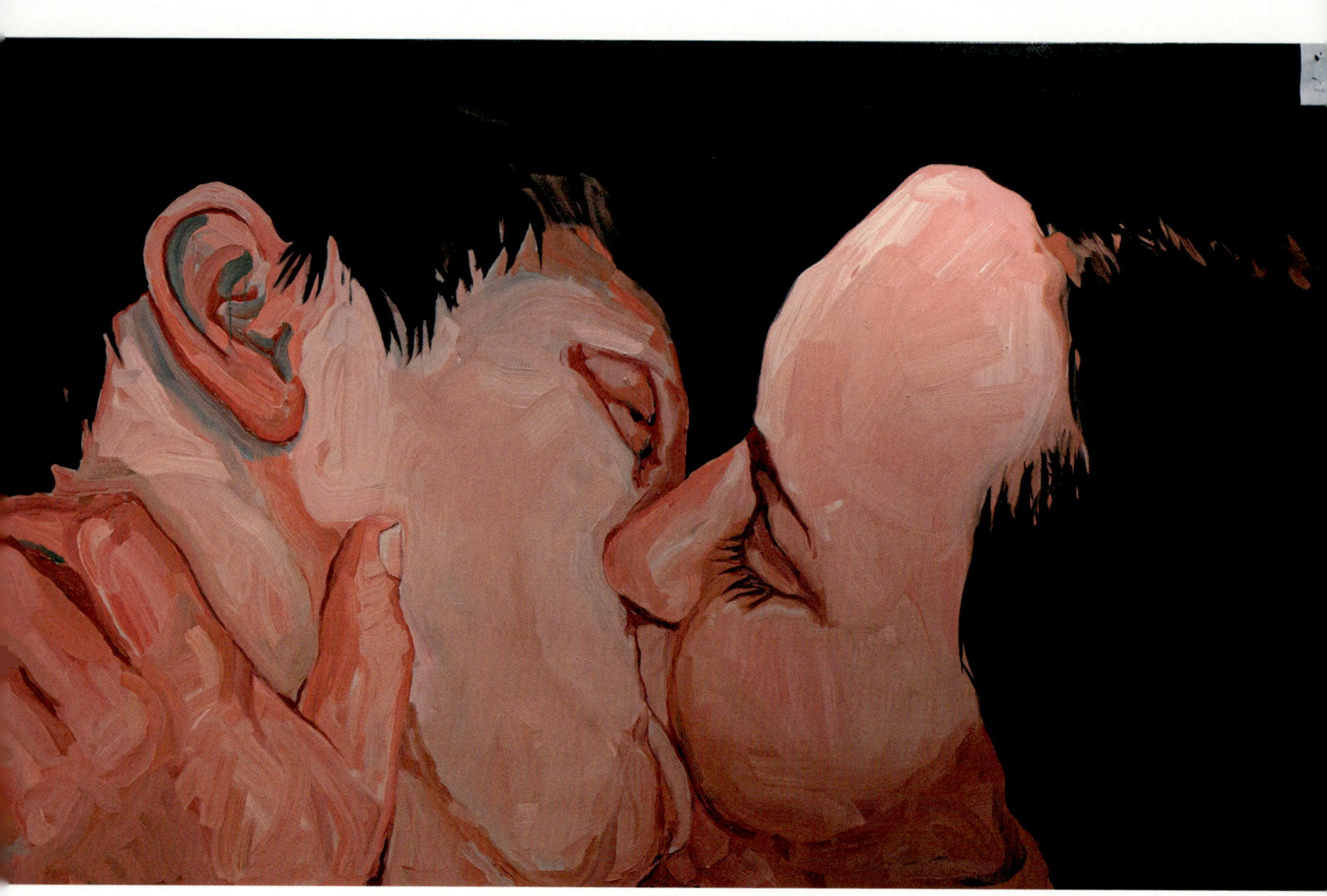

June 28: Kiss.

I have found my origin in mania. Today, alignment spinning
like a top, a roulette table landing on ALL BLACK. NONE
NUMBER.
You cannot know light without dark. Depression,

VII

Now, September 17, 2020
The garden is burning. Like some kind of changing of
the guard.

At night I fall out the window, hung in the air
by Jupiter, sifting my hands through
the rings of Saturn.
I feel back to when Candace and God
were born,
once caught far between the moon's
fallen horizon,

where Candace and I duck inside,
thunder, crashing, falling shadows,
full of sounds.

Then, rest. No more suffering because I
Know ~~You~~, mania, pure Being. I Know where
~~You~~ have gone, no more fear.

Now, no more flowers in the summer of
Vancouver Island, Fall days coming hung
with smoke from the south, west, north, east.

Maybe soon joy, some new awakening. Some
glimpse of Being.

VIII

Over and over—
awaken — in the mind hospital
— still writing my, your history —
nothing abstract — maybe I will
draw a few images.
Run through mind —
like sifting words of Dylan or
Mitchell or Ginsberg, seers that
SEE VISIONS. Maybe seeing
all the mad people put in cells
of medications that should be

illuminating the walls in our skull's mental projections.

Remembering the electric shocks.

Long did I look into you at 8 Washington, so did I Be with you at 503 Outlook, ALL SKY, MIRROR OCEAN, so do I hope to be with you now Cobble Hill, Vancouver Island.

Today, the other strife of my Being, the concealing muting of no hope takes over my breath, clogging my throat as I sit here unable to see through the smoke in my backyard, or the loss of everything in everything everywhere. One final glimpse as the web of life takes its last breaths in the void of space, slipping into Now, with no left or right, up , slip, down. Okay.

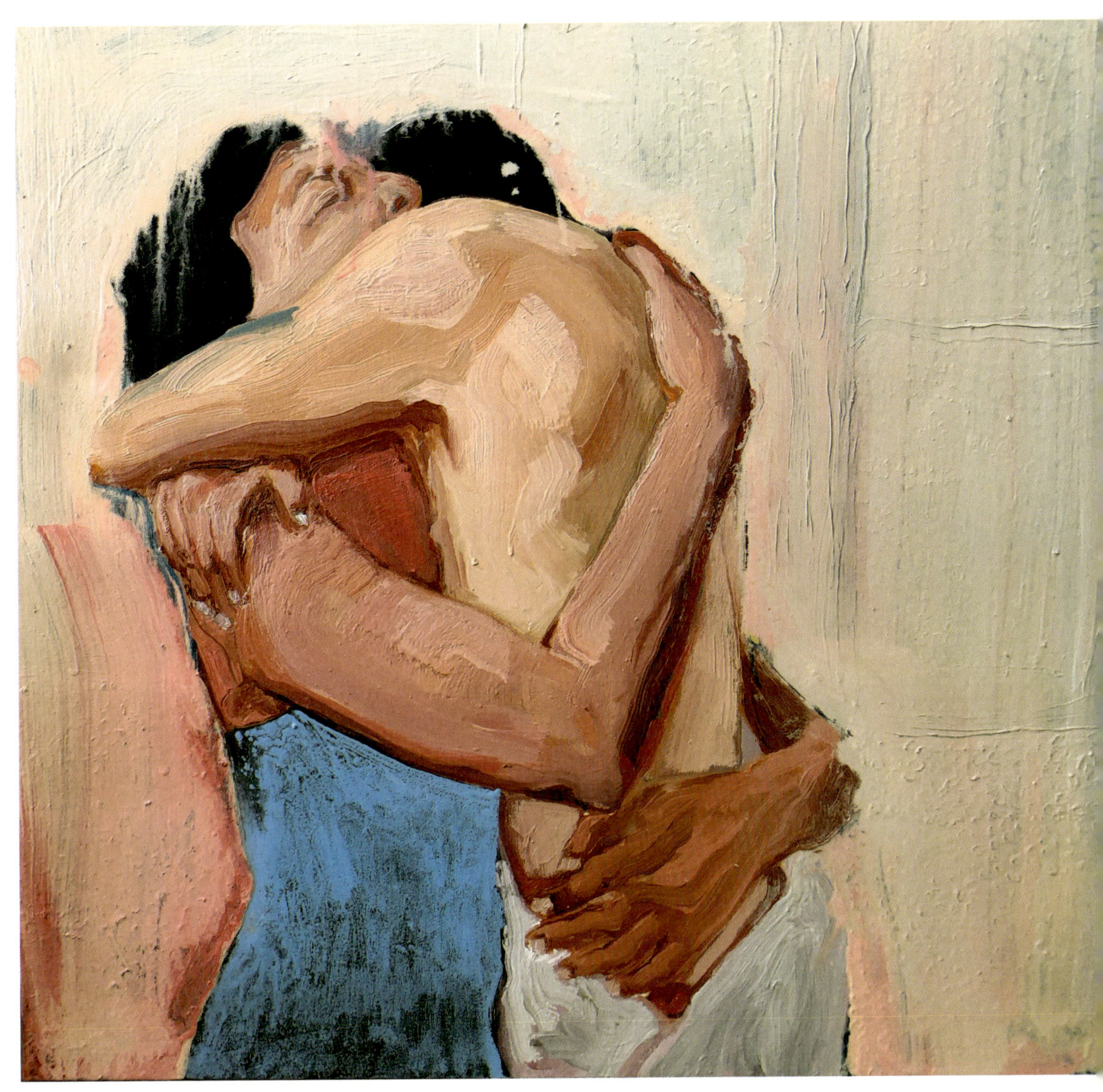

July 8: Hug.

FOR THE YOUNG GIRL NEXT TO ME, WHO IS STILL WITH ME

Spring 1991, grade one, six-years-old: intestinal attack.
UofA Hospital, seemed like months, maybe I am still in
that room.

One day, I leave my room and go to the nursing station to get a popsicle
from the freezer.
I am walking back sirens blazing nurses and
doctors running
everywhere my room || blocked off.
I turn to the room next to mine, gazing into THE portal that has opened.
The child beside me, a girl the size of a thimble, at least in my memory,
collapsing life.

The room loses structure, evaporates into a white void,
with only doctors, nurses, the small child
spotlights illuminating everything
I look to the side, into the infinite void
Mother reaching out | silent | screaming!
whatever that sound was
is gone
tears of rage
at the sacred,
reaching out
dad holding her like you do
to life.

breathe in,
breathe out

shocking
banging pressing
the hammering and hammering of fighting entropy,
hitting, clawing, resisting the fall
fighting the flow
the flow that the room became, the passing of
moment to moment
breath to breath
being to being *she* is,,, was.

Thin place. The portal is open. I am witnessing
something sacred
THE sacred
whatever that meant
to a six-year-old
thirty-six, now,
decades of pain, my kids,
her radiating in me,
forcing the dam to overflow,
antipsychotics can only conceal
so well,
sensations, a layer of tears flowing and
flowing,
transporting me into a thin place, death, O god,
Holy child
then silence, the room collapses back to form.
Death, my first death, whatever that meant to a six-year-old.

You experience these moments — after you pass across the event horizon,
a place you can't come back from, — differently through time. I thought about
it one way in an artwork in 2012. I understood it one way.
Now as a parent,
Ellie Mary
I experience it differently, the focal point moves to the mother,
tears of
~~rage~~
forgotten
sacrament
Holy
mother,
Maybe
today a cry
of layers,
I can't think about it as a parent, some things are unthinkable.

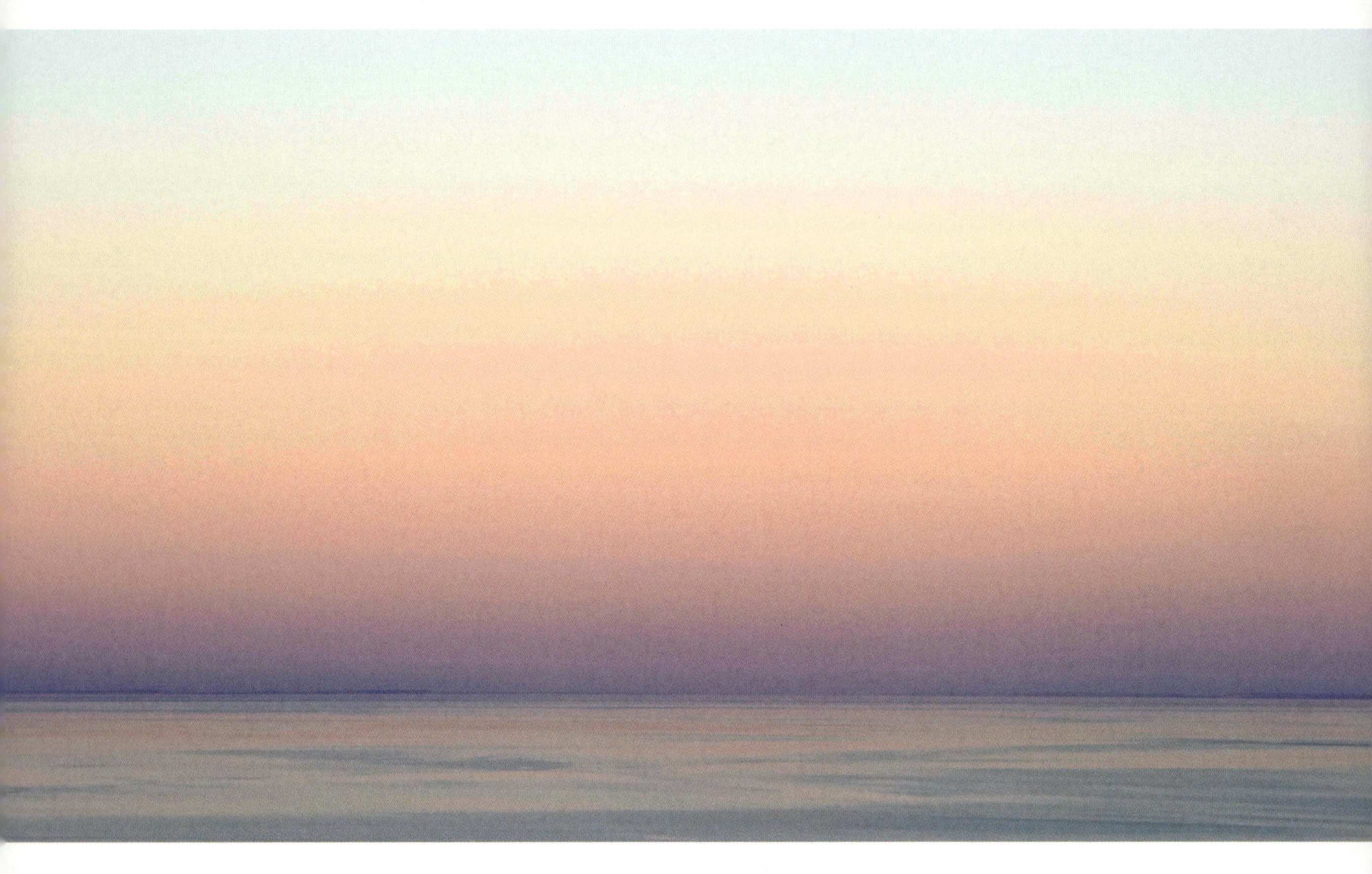

July 26. ALL SKY,
MIRROR OCEAN.

World a field within your consciousness. Grass, some trees. If you are lucky enough, flowers on the trees, preparing their vibrant fruit that begs us to world colour. Ripening as they unfold—colouring time to eat.

Do you hear that sound? A bee jumping from flower to flower, diving its head into the stamen, the petals enveloping the bee.

Have you ever seen bees without flowers or flowers without bees? They are two parts of a whole. How can we say they are separate?

Our Self is a boundary erecting being, setting up *heres* and *theres*, *insides* and *outsides*. Distinctions where there are no distinctions.

Vancouver Island: from July 18,
then,
to August 1,
now,

I record the sky gradient as the sun sets and the sky unfolds from the horizon up to the top of the world. I don't try to break up this unfolding gradient into anything separate: separate colours, or times of day, or luminosities. That would steal the sunset from what it is:

a revelation that can only be Known in its unfolding.
One becoming many—a gradient.

I am archiving this unfolding and now I will sense it. And so I sit, cross my legs, and open myself to this meditation.

I feel the ocean breeze, warm, enveloping.
I breathe in through my nose, salt yes, but sweetness as well, also the exhales of
// plants, plankton, eagles, and bees.
I feel the cushion I am resting upon and the cloud of sensation that is a body.
I sense the breath pull in ocean air, filling my lungs, lifting my body.
The exhale pours out of my nose and I can world the turbulence that flows past my lips, touching my chin.
Then again.

I sense *everything* course through my mind and body, now one, and letting drift on the ocean, opening the possibility for myself to hit the wall of the World in the boat of the Self. And I do. On July 26, I climb out. Significant. Maybe the most.

Of course, *ineffable*. Here is a field note that is never enough:

I sit at the edge of mind and slip.

A voice:

BEYOND HERE LIES NOTHING

Ancient awarenesses linger here, guides like Ovid and Dylan. Marks in the air.

I see an ocean mirror, sifting all loss and suffering.

breathe in , breathe out.

I see the sky gradient before me, in me,
purplepinkorangeyellowblue
hovering at the top of the world: a crown
Worlding a halo from the sliver of wavelengths I apprehend
And,
I am hiding from the gamma-ray bursts from faraway galaxies.

Exile. Beach sand, toes, sharp rocks. Charon is waiting, where is the coin?

breathe in
breathe out

it grows in my hand, I place it on my tongue and choke. flooding
sensations. overwhelming resistance.
clawing and beating. sand sifting between my toes and sharp rocks
pressing. terror
all directions point down.

Charon: f
a
l
l

flickering awareness: *BEYOND HERE LIES NOTHING. A land beyond the land. chillness, hostility, frozen waves of an ice-hard sea.*

don't look back. fall. okay, so I fall

sky shelf bends. heading to the hinterlands of mind, the abyss is
presenting itself:
are you ready?

raging whirlpool

mountain erodes to sand, *each grain screaming its own name*.
the sky pours and falls and I fall with it
—comets, planets, stars, galaxies.

ALL SKY. MIRROR OCEAN. Charged and rotating whirlpool.
Head barely above ocean, holding onto each breath.

The abyss pres-
ents an edge, a
limit to what I
can World. This
edge breaks
into geometric
patterns, forms
flowing in and out
of concealment,
separate yet one.
Butting up against
World.

a tsunami of awareness starts at my toes, crashes through my chest, and
blasts out the top of my head, out of mind,
universe expanding and I expand with it. Mind cracks. patterns cascade
down, through the whirlpool. awareness presses past the collapsing dome,
spreading everywhere and everywhen. pure sensory affect as I cross the event
horizon of the whirlpool,
and it just flows and flows and—

forget
~~You~~
~~Everything~~. then
HOME
Out the top of a wave,
breathe
, cresting down, then
calm.
clarity. then, flow. hear. awareness bare.

the warmth of a womb.
eons. epochs.

singularity:
the birth of a new
universe.
Unfolding.

awaken. sweet air, a breeze in my ears,
breathe in, breathe out,
water cresting at my feet, smooth everything.

now, simply,
Becoming
moment to moment
the being to being I *am*, out in the open ocean.

no-one to be alone. no-where to go. no-body.
sunbathing.
the comfort of a mother after being born.

no more waves crashing as I move up the gradient of dreaming to waking.

room to breathe.

bliss.

goodbye sweet incarnation.

I look at the ocean,
Mother Earth, sheltering.
I gaze above me,
Father Sun, giving and giving and giving. Illuminating
all.

Father Sun presses down from the sky. He is presenting Himself.
Mother Earth rises up to meet Him. She is presenting Herself.
Brighter than bright.
I do not cover my eyes as Mother Earth begins to touch Father Sun,
fusing into two infinite planes.

PURE SPACE.

my awareness begins to expand out between these planes, merging. and as I merge everywhere and everywhen becomes everything and I enter into the flow of Becoming:

ALIGNMENT.

My place in it all.

ORIGIN:
Becoming
from the birth of the universe outwards
the first stars expanding supernova, death
, the materials of life, across the cosmos,
time,
again,
again, again,
time, death, black
hole's gravity well,

Father Sun, Mother Earth, then

LIFE
organizing,
expressing itself
complexity
feeling all
the orientations,
each time lowering extropy to a miracle,
KNOWING birth,
me as a sick child normal
Candace, marriage
pain, bipolar,
pain
Elliot, pain,
Mary, mania,
VISIONS opening,
mania, opening,
psilocybin, meditation,
Styx
abyss
the open

ONE
BEING

✳ You cannot go on a journey, *here to there*, without a start to begin from, the edge to start the unfolding of a marvellous gradient to flow upon. In the beginning, there was nothing but the watery void, then light.

You cannot Know light without dark, a teaching gradation of vision outside vision: awareness. But there is no point where one ends and the other begins: zoom a little closer, look.

You cannot Know bliss without suffering, the teaching gradient of ~~You~~. *How can we say they are apart?*

You cannot Know life without death, the teaching gradient of Being. You come to Know through strife and what greater strife is there than to sleep with life and death in the same bed. The wholeness of being a being with Being.

So perfect incarnation.

To have darkness is to come to Know light, otherwise, there is nothing to see. One becomes many to come to know itself. The oldest creation story we can tell ourselves. You cannot know spontaneous life without spontaneous death: when will it happen? Now that is a strife!

Heidegger: we erect a world that sets forth an earth, and between that world and earth a strife forms and this is where Knowing is felt.

With life and death hung in the room, they pull on you as they express their origin: spontaneity. One's origin is the source of its essence. Spontaneity can only be known through its unfolding. We are after the origin. To express that origin. To live and breathe that origin. To leave before and after behind, to be a spontaneously unfolding moment to moment, breath to breath, being to being: present.

Do you sense the strife form between You and ~~You~~? The dream and the awakening. Riding that awareness of Being? To sense this strife is to come to Know. These aren't explicit knowing, but Knowing to Know. To Know death is to Know life. To *Be*.

To Know Death, teaches us how to die, which teaches us how to live. This is healing. One becomes many,

light and dark,
body and mind,
so perfect incarnation,
life and death,
to come to Know oneself. To find the origin:
alignment.

To express that alignment, reorienting to Being, moment to moment. To unconceal more than it conceals. Being a being before and within Being. To enter into the pure space of the open as no-body.

This is why we heal.

I

13.8 billions years ago, the universe is a single point, a singularity, amongst the larger flow of pure energy—Being. And all of everything, the entirety of the cosmos, held in one hot dense moment in a large primordial sea of the Greater Mind Universe.

No protons, no electrons, no forces of nature, no parts, no distinctions, no pain, no suffering, no joy, just one, just pure Being slipping outside time, no space to fill, simply infinity and eternity—all one.

And then it goes as all things go, a miracle, a quantum fluctuation, an unbelievably small blip, an unbelievably small drop in the primordial sea of the Great Mind Universe, a slipping of tectonic states, that releasing a tsunami of absolute force

—the birth of a new universe
—when ~~you~~ and ~~I~~ were born
—the epochs we share

From no time, from no space, ~~we~~ are a mystery, one radiant jewel on Indra's Net as it begins weaving itself across the unfolding expanse of Being and Time. For these first fractions of fractions of fractions of the first 10^{-36} seconds of infant time ~~we~~ split into two jewels, weaving and knotting the beginning of everything, the great expression ~~you~~ ~~II~~ continue to become, the expression that is coming to Know itself, the expression ~~you~~ inhabit now, Candace, centre of my universe, the universe I call home, the universe that makes me feel whole, sustains me, loves me. The universe that helps me, nurtures me, to express myself, to come to Know myself, moment to moment, breath to breath, being to being ~~you~~ and ~~I~~ are,

O Candace,
love of my life,
centre of everything,
beginning of everything,
crashing end to everything,
giver, shelter, home, mother.

When you are 10^{-36} seconds old the force of quantum gravity emerges yet the electromagnetic, weak, and strong nuclear forces remain one. Then, you expand 10^{25} until you are the size of a grain of sand at 10^{-32} seconds. Wow! Look at ~~you~~ unfold! ~~You~~ cool and cool as this happens, then ~~you~~ quantum tunnel to a new energy state where ~~you~~ slip down and down in energy blasting ~~you~~ to reheat back to the beginning of time. ~~You~~ continue to unfold and the forces separate and over fractions of a second ~~you~~ go through epoch after epoch as ~~you~~ become ~~you~~. The home for all of us, the Great Mother.

~~You~~ are a second old now, 10 light years across, and ~~you~~ are unfolding marvellously. In unbelievable heat ~~you~~ start to fuse with ~~yourself~~ in primordial nucleosynthesis, creating the first expressions of hydrogen, helium, and lithium, the continuing distinctions, the first separations from oneness, ~~your~~ first steps in the unbelievable unfolding as ~~you~~ Become with ~~me~~. The first primordial black holes form, quaking in ~~our~~ Being. ~~You~~ sow the seeds of everything that will take shape. Everything that will become hope, suffering, joy, love, love love love holy! love.

~~You~~ exist as a plasma, 42 million light years in size, a hot hot hot universe of protons and photons, an infant's bath, but ~~you~~ are unfolding now, unfolding across time, unfolding across space,and as ~~you~~ unfold ~~you~~ cool from infinity and after 380,000 years ~~you~~ look over a chasm

and ~~you~~ slip

from plasma to gas and release light from heaven, a light I can look at today with my own eyes, the first clear photograph of an infant ~~you~~ and ~~I~~

—the Cosmic Microwave Background.

When I look at that picture, when I look at ~~you~~, I see so few distinctions, still so uniform, still so very much one. Yet I look closer and closer and can see tiny fluxes, tiny shifts, 1 in 100,000 parts difference, and I can see the Baryon Acoustic Oscillations, the first imprints of ~~your~~ voice, that signal the beginning unfolding, the imprint of the entire universe to come, a beginning organization, the first impression of ~~your~~ larger Mind, that will collapse into the galaxies we see today, the galaxies we are made from, the galaxies we are apart of. I look at this and fall in love with this beginning unfolding, the moment to moment, flux to flux unfolding I am witnessing today in ~~you~~.

Then ~~you~~ go dark, no visible light,
darkness covers the face of the deep,
yet ~~you~~ continue to unfold and express ~~yourself~~
continue to come Know ~~yourself~~
as the winds and rivers of dark matter flow, absolute flow, the essence of flow
collecting and collecting hydrogen and helium
collecting everything along the structures ~~you~~ created with ~~your~~ voice at the beginning of time
and as ~~your~~ essence unfolds for 100 million years ~~you~~ say with it
Let there be light
And then there was light.

From the formless void   the birth of the first star
, then the next,   then the next   pull
pull
pull
then   collapse
BOOM
nuclear fusion
explosion kept in a
gravity well
balance between outer
and inner
hydrogen begets   helium
helium   lithium
burning, radiating
filling ~~you~~ with light
with warmth
then BOOM
Supernovae

the heavens become
magical fireworks   that   weave
jewel after jewel
on   Indra's Net
expanding with dark energy
making space for spaciousness
reflecting each other
and in one of those stars you and I
are born
first pebbles of

Carbon	Oxygen	Iron
all the mystery	all the chimes	all the holiness
		that will, again,
over cosmic time, epochs	over unimaginable space	we
collect in dust clouds	collapsing into a new star	breathing
solar winds	hitting some ancient	
	planet's	soul
bathing it in light	warmth	time
and	time	and
supernova	the gold in our blood,	
	rings	fused
flung into the cosmos	spreading seeds of	life
across our tiny patch	of cosmic space	star, supernova
evaporating the planet	and here you, I live a	
	lifetime	and

begin lifetimes	together in stars,	
	gas giants	and
comets, other oceans	that sit just right	where we
fuse the body with a soul	that will become our	
	home	that
grows blue and green	that unfolds the most	
	creative	expressions
that are so holy	that are so absolutely	
	outstanding	that
lower entropy to a	miracle	that
haunt the cosmos with	radiant jewels	reflecting
the whole of ~~you~~	the whole of our cosmos	in the
whites of your eye	as you look at me	as you
look at Ellie Mary	as you flow and unfold	in
this life	in all the lifetimes we	share
in this moment	in this moment	in
this moment	and you fill my lungs	that
weaves in my blood	and nourishes all of me	with
~~your~~ giving essence	from the beginning of	time
when ~~you~~ and ~~I~~	were	born.

Then, I look at another photograph of child ~~you~~. The Hubble Deep Field image looks back at the earliest you, the earliest stains and stresses of your unfolding, infant galaxies, field of galaxies, so much different than the galaxies we see today, the galaxy we sit in now, the home where I looking at you through the pane of glass, thinking about us scared for you last night, me in the emergency hospital parking lot, unable to go in with you because of COVID procedures, sending texts that are never enough, no matter the poetry, nothing can describe the centre of my universe, ~~you~~.

II

I am 12. The doctors say I might grow out of my surgeries, my side effects, my pain. They said I might be normal, I just need to unfold a bit further. I am in my new junior high school in St. Albert, Alberta, in the Canadian prairies, knowing nothing outside this weeping home.

24 years later, I have so few memories to fall into. So much lost to the march of time. I can't even remember my teacher's name or which of my friends were in my class. I do remember walking past a room, a room my memory can World the footing I am standing in,

I stand in the hall

looking into another grade 7 classroom
and I see a girl
with skin like I had never seen
with hair so blonde   so yellow
I saw a girl amongst a group of girls
none of whom stay in my memory
and that was the first time
(in this life)
I see you, my Candace
the jewel on the great net
releasing a quake in my being
Holy! Candace, Holy! Me, Holy! ~~you~~ and ~~I~~

13.8 billion years, travelling the length of the cosmos, the full expression of time, and here we are. Only a classroom apart—

III

Do you remember the hug we had in my basement 18 years ago?
18-year-old children.
I'll never forget it.   It was like coming home.   Like you and I have lived
this life a hundred
times together, and this
was another cycle. And
I am overjoyed to do it
again—
again with you.

We were two kids, no idea what we wanted in life, other than
(with unbelievable insight)
that we wanted to love each other.   And we are good at that.
Really good.

You are so full of heart,   you just love and love and love,
feel all the feels,
shed all the tears,
for you, for me.
I love that about you.   You balance me, give more and more to each experience
that I, alone,
cannot experience.   Sure we can get along solo,
sometimes,
but when we share a moment together it is a
revelation,
ecstasy,

love,
heart, home.
I am so lucky to do this, this moment to moment, breath to breath with you.
Love of my life,
centre of everything,
beginning of everything,
crashing end to everything,
giver, shelter, home, mother.

We dream.
There is no one I would rather dream with.
We are so good at falling into each other dreams,
okay, no worries,
we can do anything together.
And so we dream all the dreams of a million lifetimes together,
and each time I get to live out a lifetime with you,
in each moment,
in each breath,
and now we dream of these girls and the dreams we hope they have some day.
We dream of ocean air,
sand sifting between our toes,
sun-kissed everything,
looking out over the Pacific,
looking for an origin,
the origin of this dream,
that spills into the next,
and so the waves crest at our feet
as we prepare to fall into the next dream.
I hope we pass this onto our girls,
that they have the confidence to look at
someone,
hold someone,
love someone,
render themselves vulnerable,
open,
take my heart,
carry my heart,
I'll carry yours,
like you and I do,
because ~~you~~ and ~~I~~ are
the root of the root,
the bud of the bud,
the sky of the sky,

of the tree we call life
—and,
if we dream enough,
we will pass this to our
girls and their partners in life,
in time,
in every lifetime.

I love you Candace,

Brad

Introduction

creation-as-research

Owen Chapman and Kim Shawchuk's 2012 article "Research-Creation: Intervention, Analysis and 'Family Resemblances'" was where I encountered the term *creation-as-research* as they described four categories or "family resemblances" of research-creation:

> research-for-creation,
> research-from-creation,
> creative presentations of research, and
> *creation-as-research.*

They describe creation-as-research as "an engagement with the ontological question of what constitutes research in order to make space for creative material and process-focused research-outcomes" (p. 49).

In 2016 creation-as-research was weaving into my understandings arising from Diane Conrad and Jamie Beck's 2015 article "Towards Articulating an Arts-Based Research Paradigm: Growing Deeper." There they imagine the ontological, epistemological, and axiological implications of creating within an arts-based research paradigm (Natalie Loveless once described arts-based research and research-creation as close cousins). These ideas laid the foundation, gave me a vocabulary, and confidence for me to build my creation-as-research practice.

I learnt ideas such as

> "We suggest that an arts-based paradigm is grounded ontologically in a belief that we are all, at a fundamental level, creative and aesthetic beings in intersubjective relation with each other and our environment" (Conrad & Beck, 2015, p. 7).
>
> "Art is fundamental to our capacity to make meaning of and give value to life; human beings are fundamentally aesthetic beings" (p. 8).
>
> "Art-making is everyone's, not just the artist's, way of making special, for sharing meaning and value" (p. 9).
>
> acknowledging "the multiple and diverse ways of coming to know through creating, embodiment, feeling, intuition, and spirit" (p. 11).
>
> or suggestions that art "does not produce concepts, though it does address problems and provocations. It produces sensations, affects, intensities as its mode of addressing problems" (p. 11).
>
> arts "make space for spaciousness" (p. 12);

they often open worlds. Openings, beginnings, initiatives, new understandings, more intense these, I think, are our shared concerns. Such openings through art create a space for relationality or dialogic engagement.

And very important to me, flourishing, the sensation of pure healing:

> "An arts-based research paradigm encourages contributions towards honouring relations, human and non-human flourishing, and celebrates art's potential to transform the world" (p. 13).

Later, when I read Thomas King, Donna Haraway, and Natalie Loveless, it would only reinforce this world-transformative potential in art. Then I saw it again in all the art I co-created, all the art I created. This was like a lightning rod in Walter De Maria's sculpture *The Lightning Field*, igniting a gesture from heaven full of potential, a future, a better future.

When I was taking Diane Conrad's Arts-Based Research class in 2016, I came to *know otherwise*, awakening to what knowledge could be mined from experience: moving, sensing, noticing, pausing, witnessing, being present to the unfolding strife. That course and the scholarship we investigated filled me with curiosity, drive, spirit, and, soon to come, story.

Conversations with Natalie Loveless solidified the force of creation—the act of creation as a site for knowledge generation. What Allen Ginsberg would describe as subjective truths having an objective reality because someone has realized it—in the birth of an artwork was the birth of an artist. Natalie's text *How to Make Art at the End of the World* and our conversations have provided me with many of the concepts I used in my art and research practice to describe research-creation and related knowledge-production practices. Most importantly, it provoked me to freely create, making-special what I valued about being alive.

In 2020, reading Heidegger's "The Origin of the Work of Art" (drafted between 1935 and 1937 and first published in 1950) filled me with confidence, a bursting confidence in creation-as-research. The language of this essay changed me and filled every sentence in this book:

> *Art then is a becoming and happening of truth.* (p. 196, emphasis added)

> Truth means the essence of the true. We think this essence in recollecting the Greek word *aletheia*, the unconcealment of beings. (p. 176)

> The work-being of the work consists in the instigation of strife between the world and earth. (p. 175)

> A work, by being a work, *makes space for that spaciousness*. "To make space for" means here especially to liberate the free space of *the open region* and to establish it in its structure. This installing occurs through the erecting mentioned earlier. The work as work sets up a world. The work holds open the open region of the world. But the setting up of a world is only the first essential feature in the work-being of a work to be referred to here. (p. 170, emphasis added)

> That into which the work sets itself back and which it causes to come forth in this setting back of itself we called the earth. *Earth is that which comes forth and shelters*. Earth,

> irreducibly spontaneous, is effortless and untiring. Upon the earth and in it, historical man grounds his dwelling in the world. *In setting up a world, the work sets forth the earth.* (p. 171–72, emphasis added)
>
> World and earth are always intrinsically and essentially in conflict, belligerent by nature. Only as such do they enter into the *strife of clearing and concealing*. Setting up a world and setting forth the earth, *the work is the instigation of the strife in which the unconcealment of beings as a whole, or truth, is won.* (p. 180, emphasis added)
>
> Where this bringing forth expressly brings the openness of being, or truth, that which is brought forth is a work. Creation is such a bringing forth. (p. 187)

Creation is such a bringing forth,   supernovae,   stardust

Heidegger informed my experience of Carl Jung's 1933 *Modern Man in Search of a Soul*:

> But this question forces itself upon us as soon as we come to the visionary mode of creation. We are astonished, taken aback, confused, put on our guard or even disgusted—and we demand commentaries and explanations. We are reminded in nothing of everyday, human life, but rather of dreams, night-time fears and the dark recesses of the mind that we sometimes sense with misgiving. (p. 158)
>
> The vision is not something derived or secondary, and it is not a symptom of something else. It is true symbolic expression—that is, the expression of something existent in its own right, but imperfectly known...We need not try to determine whether the content of the vision is of a physical, psychic or metaphysical nature. In itself it has psychic reality, and this is no less real than physical reality. (p. 162)
>
> It is not alone the creator of this kind of art who is in touch with the night-side of life, but the seers, prophets, leaders and enlighteners also. However dark this nocturnal world may be, it is not wholly unfamiliar. Man has known of it from time immemorial—here, there, and everywhere; for primitive man today it is an unquestionable part of his picture of the cosmos. (p. 163)
>
> The primordial experience is the source of his creativeness; it cannot be fathomed, and therefore requires mythological imagery to give it form. (p. 164)
>
> The secret of artistic creation and of the effectiveness of art is to be found in a return to the state of participation mystique—to that level of experience at which it is man who lives, and not the individual, and at which the weal or woe of the single human being does not count, but only human existence. (p. 172)

Of course many other texts and conversations nurtured, developed my creation-as-research practice, but these were the most significant. Spending a night with friends sitting in a James Turrell work in Houston, Texas, in 2015 contributed to this just as much. Same with Brian Webb and Gary James

Joynes's dance *Liminal* in 2019. Over years, these texts weaved and knotted into my Being and Art creating a free region to create and Know

love, dissolving
merging
one

Suffering is the cause to bring about its end

This idea was an interpretation from Buddhism that kept arising from conversations over the years and was most clearly stated in Thich Nhât Ha nh's 2014 *No Mud, No Lotus:*

> We must remember that suffering is a kind of mud that we need in order to generate joy and happiness. Without suffering, there's no happiness. So we shouldn't discriminate against the mud. We have to learn how to embrace and cradle our own suffering and the suffering of the world, with a lot of tenderness. (p. 13)
>
> If you know how to make good use of the mud, you can grow beautiful lotuses. If you know how to make good use of suffering, you can produce happiness. We do need some suffering to make happiness possible. (p. 14)

Co-creating

This term is built off ideas from Anita Sinner and Diane Conrad's text *Creating Together: Participatory, Community-Based, and Collaborative Arts Practices and Scholarship across Canada* from 2015. Conrad and Sinner describe the capacity of art to generate new knowledge with "emotional and embodied qualities" (p. xiv). A mode of investigation that can lead to new insights, themes, and understandings. They describe the experience of creating together as a process involving aspects of "place, story, embodiment, health and wellbeing, and witnessing" (p. xvii). They note that, "Oftentimes, the process of creating together involves listening, seeing, attunement, and attentiveness, mindful attendance, or 'with-ness.' Such participatory practice may be described as a disposition that is rooted in humility, conviction, trust, and vulnerability on the part of the artist-collaborator and researcher" (p. xvii). In my co-creation practice, I identify deeply with this idea of witnessing based on a foundation of humility, trust, and vulnerability. By witnessing communities and co-creating art, we are listening to people's stories, their pain and hope, attuning to their understandings and questions. What we value.

Mysticism

This is not a term I would want to describe in its entirety. For me, it is meant to carry multiple, contradictory meanings that are always in flux and evolving. It will mean different things at different times for each person. The closest I will get to describing it is based on an Alan Watts's lecture where he describes it as an "ecological awareness," what I interpret as awareness to overwhelming connection and interdependence, maybe through the image of Indra's Net where the whole of everything is interdependent and reflected in every node on the great net of Being (Watts, n.d.; Unitarian Universalist Association, n.d.).

weave and knot author, subject, environment, and spirit

This book is written autoethnographically, weaving the author, subject, environment, and spirit into a larger, longer story. My autoethnographic practice was informed by several writers and explored in depth in my doctoral dissertation. I was inspired towards this direction when reading Norman Denzin's 1997 *Interpretive Ethnography: Ethnographic Practices for the 21st Century* describe the crisis of representation as a period of

> intense reflection, "messy texts"...experiments in autoethnography...ethnographic poetics...anthropological and sociological poetry...evocative and layered accounts...short stories...the "New Journalism"...performance texts...plays...ethnographic fictions, and ethnographic novels...and narratives of the self. (p. xvii)

Denzin describes ethnography as a "form of inquiry and writing that produces descriptions and accounts about the ways of life of the writer and those written about" (p. xi). He brings the act of writing and the writer into focus, with the inquirer no longer viewed as a privileged, invisible, and objective observer, but rather as actively embedded within the writing and research—where the researcher lives the research. Further, he frames reflective, messy texts as "many sited, intertextual, always open-ended, and resistant to theoretical holism, but always committed to cultural criticism" (p. 224).

Another set of influences was Carolyn Ellis, Tony Adams, and Arthur Bochner's (2011) "Autoethnography: An Overview" and Tami Spry's (2001) "Performing Autoethnography: An Embodied Methodological Praxis." Ellis and her colleagues (2011) describe autoethnography as a challenge to "canonical ways of doing research" (p. 1). Scholars using autoethnography are concerned about "producing meaningful, accessible, and evocative research grounded in personal experience, research that would sensitizes others to issues of identity politics, to experiences shrouded in silence, and to forms of representation that *deepened our capacity to empathize with people who are different than us*" (p. 2, emphasis added). As I read and reflected on the text by Ellis et al., the importance of empathy as an integral element of my artistic explorations, both by being-with-others, and as a means of creating "meaningful, accessible, and evocative research" (p. 2) representations that enhance understanding and responsiveness of others, emerged clearly for me. The "people who are different than us" who I would be researching were ill, yet I was also ill, living with numerous chronic physical and mental illnesses that would shape, and be shaped by, my experiences with others. I realized that autoethnography offered a way to write and express this relationship.

Spry's (2001) writing on autoethnography was also influential, in particular her observation that reflecting on multiple selves across multiple contexts, can, arguably, serve to "transform the authorial 'I' to an existential 'we'" (p. 711). I used my personal stories and experience as both creative inspiration and content, exploring my personal experience in relation to others, situating new relational insights in relation to the social, allowing for difficult, critical representations, narrative and visual, resisting accepted or entrenched stories, metaphors, and ways of knowing. I leaned into connections across experience, isolated and shared, relating these to a larger cultural reality. For me, it was an emancipatory process that allowed me to explore the lived experience of illness, a universal human experience, in a more layered and complex way than I had previously been able to experience.

Further, autoethnographic messy writing allowed for the nonlinear narrative to emerge—the weaving and knotting of space and time, fluid, flowing, overlapping, contradicting, contrasting, exploding, flux, awakening, dissolving, merging.

Alberta #3

This work was written from field notes for a talk at the 2017 Society for Literature, Science, and the Arts Conference at Arizona State University in Phoenix, Arizona. The emphasis on keeping track of dates and times was influenced by Allen Ginsberg's "America" (1956). This talk was revised to create the short experimental film *Alberta #3*, was adapted into a theatre play in 2018 titled *Stormshelter (Alberta #4)*, and was rewritten for this book's opening chapter.

Sections of an early draft were published in *The Muse* (no. 9, 2019, pp. 22–28), Hamilton, Ontario.

I collapsed my experiences with Derek and Luanna into a single character for this opening chapter for storytelling purposes. Later in the book, my experiences with them will be faithfully (as best possible) portrayed.

Iqaluit, Nunavut

cloud illusions

Inspiration drawn from Joni Mitchell's song "Both Sides Now" (1969) from her album *Clouds*.

beyond here lies nothing

After reading *Why Bob Dylan Matters* by Richard Thomas (2017), I found a connection between Dylan's song "Beyond Here Lies Nothin'" (2009) and a short quote from Ovid's exile letters with competing translations. The one used in the text was from a post by Roz Haddon on the website Series of Dreams from May 25, 2020, as he links Dylan's song with Ovid's poem. The line from Ovid painted a picture of the abyss, one of my first:

> BEYOND HERE LIES NOTHING.
> A land beyond the land. Chillness, hostility, frozen waves of an ice-hard sea.

Another translation from Poetry in Translation reads,

> There's nothing further than this, except frost and foes, and the sea closed by the binding cold.

For artistic purposes, the translation that ties to Dylan's work was the one used.

falling is easier than resisting

This phrase came from a description of love—falling in love—from my therapist Ryan: falling, dissolving, merging, and entering into the larger flow as one. Part of the cresting sensation of falling in love is the resistance, holding onto the edge before the abyss, and the ecstasy comes when you quit resisting and just fall. Love—one, absolute connection, growing closer—is central to the process of healing as you leave being an individual and become *we*.

I was also learning about falling in psychedelic experiences. Inclinations from Timothy Leary, Ram Dass, and Ralph Metzner's *The Psychedelic Experience: A Manual Based on the Tibetan Book of the Dead* (2007) in relation to ego-death.

Also found in The Beatles 1966 song "Tomorrow Never Knows," where John Lennon sings about how surrendering to the void isn't death or leaving but rather, Being, Knowing, believing, and a new beginning.

Telling Stories Otherwise

stories

Natalie Loveless changed my life, helped me re-story my research and the life that encompasses it, with her 2019 book *How to Make Art at the End of the World: A Manifesto for Research-Creation*, where she writes, "Stories are powerful. The stories that we believe, the stories that we live into shape our daily practices, from moment to moment. They have the power to promise some futures and conceal others. They encourage us to see some things and not others" (p. 20). I continue to breathe that statement like a mantra.

Thomas King's story from *The Truth about Stories* from 2003 opened me further to the importance of stories when he said, "Want a different ethic? Tell a different story" (p. 164).

Then Donna Haraway in her 2016 book *Staying with the Trouble* connects my evolving understandings of worlds and stories by saying, "It matters what stories make worlds, what worlds make stories" (p. 12).

Later, Sara Ahmed's 2010 *The Promise of Happiness:* "It matters, how we assemble things, how we put things together. Our archives are assembled out of encounters, taking form as a memory trace of where we have been" (p. 19).

All of these ideas connected my evolving understandings around stories and worlds, that stories had the power to transform our world. Art creates worlds. Stories are powerful.

Creating new stories, bringing stories to life, illuminating stories we don't always want to know or hear, can help to expand the boundaries of our worlds, allowing our stories to take new shapes, kindships, and loves.

—all the way down

This phrase is pulling from Donna Haraway's work on stories in *Staying with the Trouble* (2016). It is also a reference to Thomas King's *The Truth about Stories* (2003) where he speaks about a creation story of turtles all the way down. It's a beautiful image.

It's yours. Do with it what you will.

This is a direct quote from King's *The Truth about Stories* (2003, p. 119). It creates an ethic about being the listener of a story. This book will be a set of stories. *Do with it what you will.*

abyss

The idea of an exchange with the abyss came after reading Friedrich Nietzsche's *Beyond Good and Evil* (1886). The line "whoever fights with monsters should see to it that he does not become a monster in the process. And when you gaze long into an abyss the abyss also gazes into you" (1998, p. 89).

Further, I was also influenced by Timothy Morton's account of the abyss in *Hyperobjects: Philosophy and Ecology after the End of the World* (2013), where he describes the abyss as that which "allows things to co-exist: it is the nonspatial 'betweenness' of things. The abyss opens up in the interaction of any two or more objects" (p. 79). And "the abyss is not an empty container, but rather a surging crowd of beings" (p. 80).

These descriptions of the abyss painted a picture of a vast space, a psychic landscape, immense, occluded by not unknowable, inhabitable by beings for exchange: a site we could learn new ways to Be, new orientations to Being, filled with all the generations past and all the generations yet to be born, *and all of everything.*

Being

My investigation into Being began with Martin Heidegger's *Being and Time* (1927) but was most heavily influenced by his essay "The Origin of the Work of Art" (1950). That essay was very significant in opening me to the potential art had to serious philosophical inquiry: truth. His use of language, such as the words *world* and *earth*, *concealing* and *unconcealing*, *strife*, *Being*, *truth*, reoriented me to a new way to knowing through art. However, its largest influence was opening me to Eastern understandings of Being, something Heidegger notes that Western philosophy had ignored, but was a central subject in Eastern thought.

The question of Being opened me to Buddhism, Hinduism's Brahman, and Taoism where much of the book creatively expressed the ideas I was exploring there. The below texts were central to my understanding of these spiritual forms.

> Thích Nhât Hạnh's 2014 *No Mud, No Lotus: The Art of Transforming Suffering*, 2012 *Love Letter to the Earth*, and 2002 *No Death, No Fear: Comforting Wisdom for Life.*
>
> Ram Dass's 1971 *Be Here Now.*
>
> Shunryu Suzuki's 1970 *Zen Mind, Beginner's Mind.*
>
> Lao Tzu's sixth-century BCE *Tao Te Ching.*
>
> Alan Watts's 1957 *Way of Zen* and 1975 *Tao: The Watercourse Way.*

Alan Watts's recorded lectures played a large role, along with my developing practice of meditation. Further, my research into psychedelic-assisted therapy and the neuroscience and phenomenological accounts solidified my understanding of Being. Those references will come later in the bibliography.

Conversations I've had with artist and filmmaker aAron Munson since 2019 helped put all of these ideas together.

spaciousness

Diane Conrad and Jamie Beck's "Towards Articulating an Arts-Based Research Paradigm: Growing Deeper" (2015) introduced me to Heidegger's "The Origin of the Work of Art" through their nod to Heidegger when stating "art makes space for spaciousness." It took many years, but this led to Heidegger and, during this period, I experienced phenomenological accounts of spaciousness in my mediation practice. As I began to meditate with my work, in particular the work Gary James Joynes and I continue to make (*Joshua Tree* (2019–2020), *Avatar's Dream* (2019–2021), *Kingdom of Illumination* (2019–2022), *The End of the World* (2020), *The Birth of the World* (2020–2021), and *Of*

Dreaming (2023)), I *felt* the world and earth in a work of art. It opened me to a new way to Knowing, and I experienced the unconcealment of Being, an ecstatic glimpse behind the curtain of which an ordered world is painted. The abyss.

nonrational, nonlinguistic, nonlinear, with layered meanings, in flux, and on the verge of disintegration
This list is influenced by my reading of Alexis Shotwell's *Knowing Otherwise* (2011) where she cites Deborah Gould (2009), who writes, "affect is unfixed, unstructured, noncoherent, and nonlinguistic" (p. 22). This affective knowledge described by Gould and Shotwell resonated with my readings of Carl Jung and my recent research into psychedelic theory and meditation.

It may bathe you in love or wound you in hatred
Summoning Bob Dylan's 1962 "A Hard Rain's A-Gonna Fall."

In October 2020, I was thinking about sitting in a James Turrell work at Rice University in Houston, Texas, with my friends, now listening to "A Hard Rain's A-Gonna Fall," looking out my window, and I wrote this poem:

> November 2015: I am sitting with Ali Nickerson, Kyle Terrence, Emilie St. Hilaire, and Maria Whiteman in a James Turrell work at Rice University in Houston. Before: we walk across the campus, fall into hidden bars, laugh at baseball fields, take pictures in front of a slab of the Berlin Wall, and think how insane this all is.
>
> *(As we walk away, I look over my shoulder at the slab of cement and it speaks to some ancient space in me like a monolith from somewhere unknown. I did not yet understand that sensation.)*
>
> It is a warm Texan night—Caribbean winds, Live Oak trees *bent back by a hurricane breeze,* with a bottle of bourbon being passed around. Maria has Henry Flynt's "Blue Sky, Highway, and Thyme" playing on repeat on her phone; a hymn echoing around the World Turrell had erected. And between the World and Earth a strife forms that unconceals Being: Knowing. Unknown to me yet but is there, presenting itself, enveloping me. A brave new World. I open myself to the world, and the World comes in.
>
> I sink into Turrell's Earth. In my mind, we are in a large marble room, sitting on marble benches, looking at a diffuse ceiling forty feet in the air, out the cut out square, a portal to heaven. Soft LED lights bounce around in the space above. It appears immense, like some pantheon the Greeks would have debated democracy and slaves. I have my arm around Ali as we talk about the years completing our MFAs together. Me 2011, Ali and Emilie 2012, and Kyle 2013, all learning with Maria. It was like coming home.
>
> Flynt's guitar hums, his voice hums, and the space fills with presence and begins to present itself.
>
> The ceiling glows gradient,
> magenta
> pink
> yellow
> teal
> everything, anything
> cut-out sky, black,   but almost purple.
> Eyes bending with mind.

The hymn continues
bouncing and filling the air
and *we* slip.
we pass the bourbon like communion
and are enveloped by the tropical air,
an Alberta winter a three hour plane ride up,
but here: shorts, t-shirts, and warmth.
Kyle, Emilie, and Maria talk, but
Ali and I sit together. She is a visionary artist
who doesn't make art anymore.
Earlier we were at the Rothko Chapel. Natalie was there too.
I don't think it resonates in her.
But I look up and up, black, black,
pain.
This is the pain ~~I~~ knew,
know.
Hello, Rothko.
I didn't yet meditate, but sitting there
I look up and up,
then down and
down.
I sit on these benches
cross my legs
and scan those images.
BLACK COLOUR
NONE NUMBER.
Sure. Okay.
I can go there with you, Rothko. Mark.
depression,
then,
suicide.
release
he paints
pure affective
experience
full of
mythical battles
soldiers, angels
saints, priests
stacking block
on black on block
fuzzing gaze
lens shifting
the edges, back
to
the beginning of
Mind,

the ancient
cathedral, where
we sing hymns of
souls and bodies
fused on the plains
of Africa, weaving
Indra's netting
to catch the universe
to reflect the Greater
Mind back onto itself

We leave and the sky is blue, bluer than it was before,
that chapel changed the threshold. Changing something
in
me.
We walk down the street into another building. This time
Janet Cardiff and George Bures Miller.
Room black,
Sound lost to memory and time. But full presence.
Mirrors hanging and spinning.
My mind turns back to 2010, Cardiff and Miller, before,
Art Gallery of Alberta.
A Japanese room in a storm,
Storm Room
and *The Murder of Crows,*
sound in a way I never knew possible,
waiting for alignment.
October 17, 2020,
I walk downstairs from watching and
listening to Gary and my first full draft of
Kingdom of Illumination. Scale and sound
placed in my imagination sometime ago.
Working on it for the past fifteen months.
Now almost done.
Whirlpools rage, ocean at the beginning of
time, *before God and Candace were born,*
Sun presents itself.
Sunrise split like the paintings at the chapel,
standing vertical.
Portal open. No fear, I created this for this moment.
Okay
I'll pass through.
I've never seen all the videos together.
Waiting for alignment.
the right time to allow it to unfold.

I have fashioned a web. A web to
catch my inner universe. Droplets
collect on the web and I see myself
fusing with Gary, fusing with the
room, the clouds outside, the tectonic
plates of Juan de Fuca and Pacific
preparing for a tsunami of force and
time, and that swells in my mind and
out of my mind.

My mind pulls out of 2010, then out from earlier today,
and I am with Turrell, with Ali, with Flynt,
and the guitar hammers and hammers,
fingers,   nails,   strings,
resonating in the body of the guitar,
resonating in Flynt's mouth,
resonating in my ears, body, mind.
Reflecting in all the
jewels
resonating as one on Indra's Net, the net of
jewels,
the
jewels
spilling down from the waterfall playing in front of
me: *Kingdom of Illumination.*

And as I sit there, and I sit here, now, I fuse with Dylan's
Hard Rain
— just a hard rain:
What will I do now?
Present with Turrell, with Ali, fusing in jewels,
thinking of his, her visions, memories—
I look out and the rain is a falling—Salt Spring
Island not visible, for now—so much life
growing and growing here.
Dreaming of Avatar Grove, just two hours away,
west coast, green everything, red-brown
soil,
the Dreamtime of that forest.
To get there I drive through Cowichan Indian
Reserve 9, where the flowers are all empty.
Before, I turn on the news and see Neskantaga First
Nation, still!, without water. Poisoning
floods of no-sense.

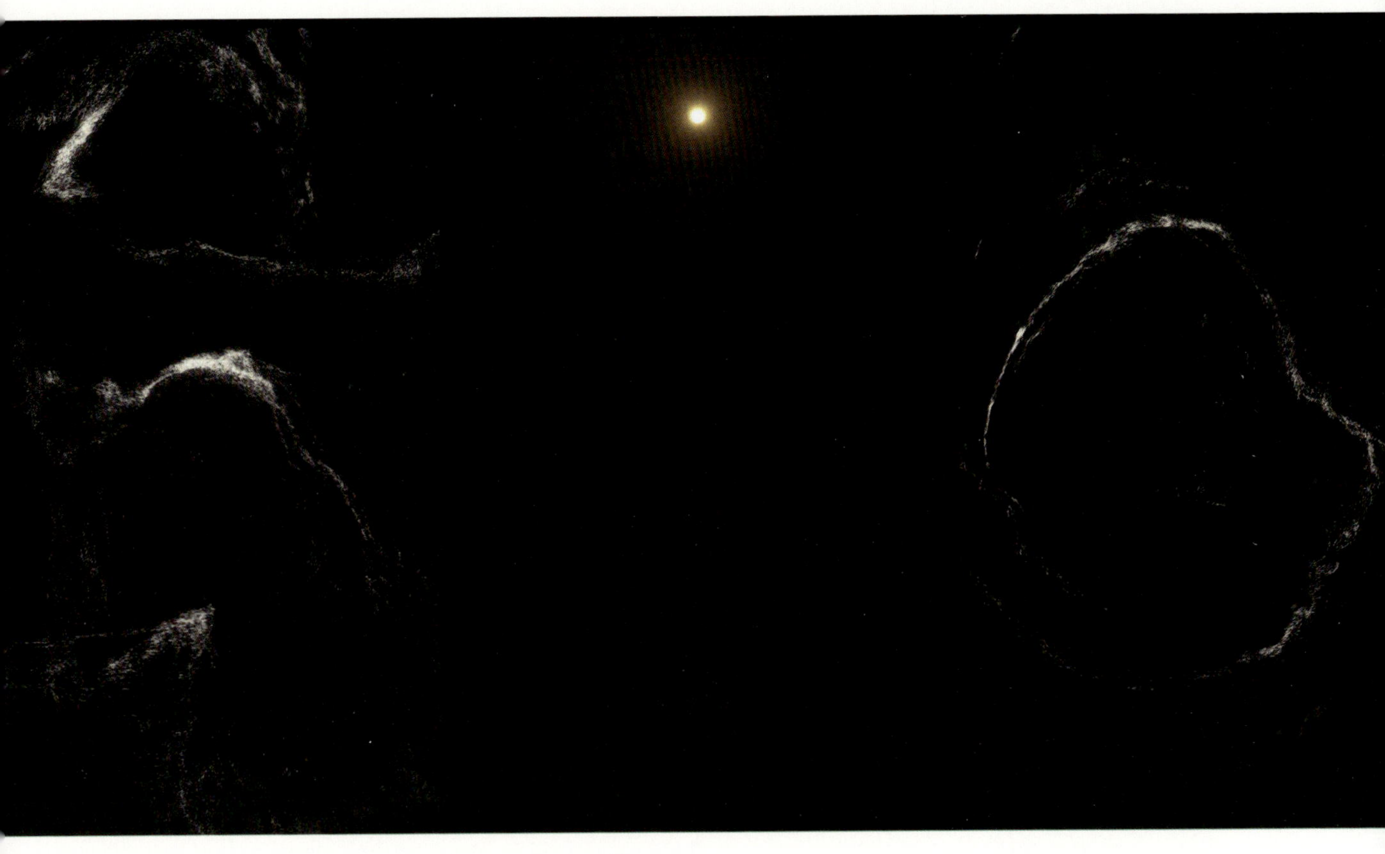

Kingdom of Illumination (the abyss), 2020–2021. 3 of 8 films. Created with Gary James Joynes.

Or, as I sit in the Cowichan Valley talking to
professors as Santa Cruz burns about
the philosophy of prisoners in San Quentin.
Thinking of all the men that put them there.
Or, the fires of Mi'kmaq fishers. Mad, desperate
Nova Scotia, some Canada's
executioners,
whose faces are ALWAYS well hidden.
Or, I turn bleak and weak and then angry, resentful,
fighting with family and friends, strangers,
PHANTOMS, VISIONS, begging for a future
for you or me, Ellie / Mary, or hope, some
time without hunger, the memory of the
souls filling me and you and the trees
listening in Avatar's Dream.
BLACK COLOUR, NONE NUMBER
And with all this madness, this pain, I open myself,
even if for a moment, some time where I am
not my Self, and I am ~~ME~~, or ~~YOU~~
and we merge, one, and with our
breath we tell it
speak it
think it
breathe it.
And then I am the vision, and you are the vision,
standing on the mountains of Moses or
under the Bodhi tree of a Buddha, putting
our hand on the ground, AND flowers
spring forth, bathing the world in colour,
sending scents into our nose, and into our
mind, and we crack open, AWAKEN,
presenting, reflecting me, you, to everyone,
everywhere, and everywhen.
And then I stand in the sands of Mystic Beach,
breathing the name of each grain like a
mantra, no longer alone, watching the
waves crash, looking into the distance
waiting for a tsunami, and I take off my
shoes, forget my clothes, and walk out into
the ocean, forsaken warmth, feeling the ebb
and flow that is water, an essence, and with
that essence I look towards an origin.
And at my origin maybe I'll sing, sing songs to
Ellie and Mary at bedtime, mostly a Case of
You, hoping I'm as constant as a Northern
Star, drawing maps of Canada with Ellie
Mary,

O, Canada

O Ellie, asking for "One Too Many
Mornings," the song we have sang together
for your lifetime, our lifetimes, that reminds
me we have been doing this across time, no
matter the beginning or pressing ending,
sensing everything between my toes and
yours   Ellie   Mary. Candace , Holy!
And it's Hard, it's a hard, a hard rain is a falling.

visionary art, primordial images, and the abyss

Each of these are terms from Carl Jung, used in *Modern Man in Search of a Soul* (1933), written closely to when Heidegger wrote "The Origin of the Work of Art" (1935–1937), and I felt an immense connection between these works. The following quote from Jung was incredibly influential in the shaping of the text's central ideas around visionary art and the abyss/unconscious:

> [Artistic expression] is a strange something that derives its existence from the hinterland of man's mind—that suggests the abyss of time separating us from pre-human ages, or evokes a super-human world of contrasting light and darkness. It is a primordial experience which surpasses man's understanding, and to which he is therefore in danger of succumbing. The value and the force of the experience are given by its enormity. It arises from timeless depths; it is foreign and cold, many-sided, demonic and grotesque. A grimly ridiculous sample of the external chaos...it bursts asunder our human standards of value and aesthetic form. The disturbing vision of monstrous and meaningless happenings that in every way exceed the grasp of human feeling and comprehension make quite other demands upon the powers of the artist than do the experiences of the foreground of life. These never rend the curtain that veils the cosmos; they never transcend the bound of humanly possible, and for this reason are readily shaped to the demands of art, no matter how great a shock to the individual they may be. But the primordial experiences rend from top to bottom the curtain upon which is painted the picture of an ordered world, and allow a glimpse into the unfathomed abyss of what has not yet become. Is it a vision of other worlds, or of the obscuration of the spirit, or of the beginning of things before the age of man, or of the unborn generations of the future? We cannot say that it is any or none of these. (pp. 156–57)

Much of this section is weaving and knotting Nietzsche, Haraway, Loveless, Shotwell, Morton, Heidegger, Jung, Watts, Nhât Hạnh, and Suzuki together in preparation for the central exploration of the text: Being, visionary art, and healing.

Edmonton, Alberta

This work was first exhibited in the *FLUX* exhibition at dc3 Art Projects in Edmonton, Alberta, in January 2017.

origin

This is from Heidegger's "The Origin of the Work of Art" where he notes that "The origin of the work of art—that is, the origin of both the creators and the preservers, which is to say of people's historical existence—is art. This is so because art is in its essence an origin: a distinctive way in which truth comes into being, that is, becomes historical" (2008, p. 202). *The origin is the source of one's essence.* This was a great provocation that opens more than it conceals.

Cancer

war metaphors

Influenced by Susan Sontag's 1979 *Illness as Metaphor*, where she investigates the patterns of metaphor used to describe illness, focusing on tuberculosis in the nineteenth century and cancer in the twentieth. She points out how "the controlling metaphors in descriptions of cancer are, in fact, drawn...from the language of warfare: every physician and every attentive patient is familiar with, if perhaps inured to, this military terminology" (p. 64). The broader connection I see in her work is the importance placed upon the kinds of stories that we tell ourselves about illness, the types of linguistic moves we make to narrate illness to ourselves: as with Haraway's work, we can see here how much it matters what stories we use to explain our worlds.

and all of everything

This is the conceptual title for by current body of film work—the guiding light. The first was a ten-minute silent work that was part of the *Processor* exhibition at the Art Gallery of Alberta in summer 2019. Later *Joshua Tree* and *Avatar's Dream* would add to it, created with Gary James Joynes—more continue to spill out. In December 2018, I was reading Barry Miles's *Allen Ginsberg: Beat Poet* from 2010 and immersing myself in Ginsberg's *Howl* from 1956. During my first psilocybin experience, I wrote in the back of that book, "To Elliot and Mary, Every artwork is your philosophy of everything at the moment. And all of everything. Love, Dad."

I was writing to them, dreaming of all the expressions and creativity I hope for them in their life. How when you create a world, and it brings forth an earth that shelters, that the fullness of what you are living and breathing, what you value, what you value about being alive, is imprinted in the betweenness of the world and earth, in the strife, that releases a quake in your Being. A revelation on Indra's Net, reflecting everything from your inner universe—a subjective truth given objective reality because you have realized it in a work of art, and in that moment you find your origin.

I was also thinking about the work I would make next month: *And All of Everything.* It was a meditation on stillness, the march of time, and the growing sense of being out of time. All the things that would begin to develop in my meditation practice starting in June 2019 after meeting aAron. At that moment, *And All of Everything* was my philosophy of everything, like *Howl* was the full summation of everything Ginsberg felt, sensed, experienced, believed, wept to and for.

A Research Meeting

Otherworlds

This idea of the Otherworld comes from Aldous Huxley's *The Doors of Perception* from 1954 and *Heaven and Hell* from 1956. Ginsberg was my first connection back to William Blake (*Howl* and these texts were written at the same time in the 1950s), but these texts were my second glance back to Blake visions and mysticism. Both Ginsberg and Huxley were links towards the connections between art, spirituality, illumination, and psychedelics.

Being

a description is not absolute Being

Many years ago, I remember reading this translation of the Tao first in Lao Tzu's *Tao Te Ching:* "The Tao that can be understood is not the eternal, cosmic Tao." Then I read Alan Watts's *Tao: The Watercourse Way* from 1975, where there is a list of translations:

> The Tao which can be spoken of is not the eternal Tao.
> The Tao that can be told of is not the Absolute Tao.
> The Way that can be told of is not an Unvarying Way.
> The Tao that is the subject of discussion is not the true Tao.
> The Way that may truly be regarded as the Way is other than a permanent way.
> The Flow that can be followed is not the eternal Flow.
> The Course that can be discoursed is not the eternal Course.
> The Force that is forced isn't true Force.
> The Tao that can be tao-ed is not the invariable Tao. (p. 39)

the unconcealmet of Being

This is an idea from Heidegger's "The Origin of the Work of Art" about how experiencing art, the strife between World and Earth, can reveal a glimpse at truth: the unconcealment of Being.

becoming, enlightenment, individuation, and self-actualization

These states of Being are where art becomes so important for healing. I believe all art is the act of healing and is a fallen field note from that activity. But we must broaden our experience of healing. We are not just healing from a physical or mental illness. Nor are we healing from a physical or mental trauma, one that has an experiential moment. Yes, it *can* be those, but it *can* be more than that. We are all suffering. Buddha noted that. Nietzsche noted that. This is an ancient and universal experience. Buddha says that suffering is the cause to bring about its end. Nietzsche notes that suffering pushes us to grow, personally, collectively, spiritually. Suffering is what helps us go from *here* to *there*. For Buddha, this was the path to enlightenment. For Nietzsche, this was to become the *overman: becoming*. For Jung, this was *Individuation*, a wholeness between your conscious and unconscious world and completion of Self. For Maslow, this was *self-actualization*, the full realization of your being, peak experience. For me, this is life's expression *to grow closer*. All of these are healing journeys.

column of air

This image came from Allen Ginsberg speaking about Bob Dylan in *No Direction Home* from 2005 where he says,

> What struck me was that he had become one—or had become identical with his breath. Dylan had become a column of air, so to speak, at certain moments, where his total physical and mental focus was this single breath coming out of his body. He had found a way in public to be almost like a shaman, with all of his intelligence and consciousness focused on his breath.

This state of Being was about absolute flow, summoning force, dissolving.

Later in the film, Ginsberg gives one of his most influential statements on art: "Poetry is words that are empowered that make your hair stand on end, that you recognize instantly as being some form of subjective truth that has an objective reality to it because somebody's realized it—Then you call it poetry later."

laying like a trap, a trap that keeps you from bathing in the open

Giorgio Agamben has an amazing interpretation of Heidegger in *The Open: Man and Animal* from 2004 where he describes the tension between man and animal and their relationship to the open. He then notes that the human's "eyes have instead been 'turned backward' and placed 'like traps' around him. While man always has the world before him—always only stands 'facing opposite' and never enters the 'pure space' of the outside—the animal instead moves in the open, in a "nowhere without the no'" (p. 57).

Healing

to keep life expressing we heal...

Sha shared this idea with me from his friend Ebon Fisher.

Default-Mode Network

My interpretation of the Default-Mode Network in relation to the self, story, and altered states of consciousness comes the Robin Carhart-Harris et al.'s 2014 article "The Entropic Brain: A Theory of Conscious States Informed by Neuroimaging Research with Psychedelic Drugs" in *Frontiers in Human Neuroscience*.

Indra's Net

The first time I encountered the idea of Indra's Net was from "Episode Five: Annihilation of Joy" from *Midnight Gospel* (2020). This was the beginning of my sustained mediation on Buddhism and immediately resonated with something primordial in my being. It was fleshed out from Alan Watts's four lectures titled *The Net of Jewels* and my ongoing conversations with aAron Munson.

worlding me in foot

This phrase was an idea of weaving Heidegger's (through Agamben's *The Open*) and Jakob von Uexküll's (*A Foray into the Worlds of Animals and Humans*, 2010) idea of *worlding worlds* with the quantum mechanics concept of collapsing a wave function, a superposition of many possible states, into one state through observation. I observe the moon and collapse its wave function that permeates the entire universe into the gravity well it sits in space, and it observes me and collapses my wave function permeating the entire universe to this footing I find myself in.

Stories and Worlds

In 2018 Dan Harvey and I co-wrote a book chapter called "'Like Watching a Movie': Notes on the Possibilities of Art in the Anthropocene" (published in *Interrogating the Anthropocene: Ecology, Aesthetics, Pedagogy, and the Future in Question*) that builds on Haraway's stories. Writing this chapter was my first encounter with Haraway's ideas on the scale of stories. We write of Haraway,

> The scale of the stories we tell ourselves matters: too big, and they can overwhelm us, breeding fatalism and nihilistic self-destruction; too small, and they seem unimportant, and can just as easily breed either acceptance or ignorance, neither of which seem likely to generate action. We need stories that are "just big enough to gather up the complexities and keep the edges open and greedy for surprising new and old connections" (Haraway 2015: 160). (Necyk & Harvey, 2018, p. 240)

I was filled with hope when Haraway writes in 2016's "Tentacular Thinking," "Revolt needs other forms of action and other stories for solace, inspiration, and effectiveness," and, "There are so many good stories yet to tell, so many netbags yet to string, and not just by human beings."

I began storying otherwise with these thinkers:

> Donna Haraway's 2003 *The Companion Species Manifesto*; her 2016 "Tentacular Thinking" in *e-flux*, and her 2016 *Staying with the Trouble* .
>
> Thomas King's 2003 *The Truth about Stories.*
>
> Natalie Loveless's 2019 *How to Make Art at the End of the World.*.

Worlding

Giorgio Agamben's 2004 *The Open* was my first introduction to Uexküll and Heidegger (immediately after I read Uexküll's *A Foray into the World of Animals and Humans*, 2010). The idea of worlding, the world-making capacity of our body and mind, was like some kind of changing of the guards. It was part spiritual, which I didn't understand back in 2011, like each person, tree, grain of sand was a Buddha, a god in its own way, a world-generating being—and from the formless void there was light. I found Heidegger's idea of a wordless stone or the poor in world animal terribly anthropocentric and dated, but his exploration into worlding very illuminating.

When I began my meditation practice years later, I would see how thoughts and sensations would manifest within the field of consciousness; they filled my consciousness with worlds.

But worlding also resonated with my understandings of psychology and neuroscience. Yes (probably), there is a world out-there, some ultimate reality, but it might be nothing like the world in-here, within my consciousness in a mind and body, my *Umwelt*—my own perceptual world, my home. Understanding that idea isn't something the intellect can do. Sure, you can understand all the moving parts, the eye, the occipital cortex, all the small regions correlating to conscious experiences: building piece by piece our world. But to not think but *Know* takes a journey—a journey that is there for every being.

I first saw Donald Hoffman's (2015) TED talk in late 2019, and it only reinforced these ideas and gave me even more confidence in them. But it also gave me the confidence I was searching for in Buddhism. The Copernican idea that consciousness is fundamental and that we might be able to scientifically explore that idea took it solely from the realm of mysticism and rooted it in my intellectual training. I then read Hoffman's 2019 text *The Case against Reality: Why Evolution Hid the Truth from Our Eyes*, which is a sustained mediation on the fallibility of our senses and how our mind and body generates the world we inhabit. It took Uexküll, Heidegger, Agamben, the Buddha and put them all together in my mind. Hoffman will continue as a guiding light with his countless interviews and lectures.

like every grain of sand has its own name

This phrase was influenced by Bob Dylan's 1981 song "Every Grain of Sand," where the scale of this cosmic accounting resonated with the Buddha Nature in every being, person, tree, or grain of sand. It made me think there are more stars in our universe than all the grains of sand on Earth. It also resonated with Hoffman's idea of conscious agents, that everything is conscious.

Thích Nhât Hạnh explores the concept of the Buddha Nature in his *Love Letter to the Earth*, where he writes,

> In Buddhism, we say every sentient being has the ability to be awakened, and to understand deeply. We call this Buddha Nature. The deer, the dog, the cat, the squirrel, and the bird all have Buddha Nature. But what about inanimate species: the pine tree in our front yard, the grass, or the flowers? As part of our living Mother Earth, these species also have Buddha Nature. (2012, p. 18)

It promises some worlds and conceals others. You see some things and not others.

This line refers back to Natalie Loveless's (2019) descriptions of stories and worlds.

the open

This is one of those ideas beyond the linear line of word. It is an *image* as Alan Watts would say. It is spatial and nonspatial, maybe closest to *betweenness*. For me, the closest experience I have to it comes when I am immersed in a work of art (for me *Joshua Tree*), meditating, or experiencing with psilocybin. It is a free region, outside self, ego, story. Where you become a mirror that holds onto nothing, a column of air. It is a reorientation, a clearing to be with and within Being. It is a spiritual space. Not about explanation but exploration. Awakening. Openness.

the hard problem of consciousness

In his Institute of Art and Ideas talk, Donald Hoffman (2019) says the hard problem is this:

> We have a lot of interesting data that gives us correlations between certain kinds of brain activity and certain conscious experiences we have...So there is this very interesting correlation between interference with neural activity...and loss of certain kinds of conscious experience...In the science of cognitive neuroscience we have discovered scores, maybe hundreds of these kinds of correlations. Correlations are the raw data, this brain activity is correlated with that conscious experience...Correlations are not a theory. It's hard to go from correlations to a genuine theory of what's causing it. Another counterexample is, if you look at a train station, a bunch of people assemble at the train station and a few minutes later a train appears. Did the people coming to the train station cause the train to appear? No. Even though the correlation is tight—every time a group of people appears a train appears a few minutes later—is not the case that the people appearing caused the train to appear. There is some third entity—namely, a train schedule—that is coordinating both. The problem we have in the hard problem of consciousness is this: scientists have gotten hundreds of these tight correlations, we do not have a theory. We cannot explain why neural activity is correlated with conscious experiences.

thin places

In his 2012 *New York Times* article "Where Heaven and Earth Come Closer," Eric Weiner offers excellent description of thin places:

> They are locales where the distance between heaven and earth collapses and we're able to catch glimpses of the divine, or the transcendent or, as I like to think of it, the Infinite Whatever.
>
> Travel to thin places does not necessarily lead to anything as grandiose as a "spiritual breakthrough," whatever that means, but it does disorient. It confuses. We lose our bearings, and find new ones. Or not. Either way, we are jolted out of old ways of seeing the world, and therein lies the transformative magic of travel.

the journey, unfolding

The Open

the stone is wordless; the animal is poor in world; and man is world-forming

These are Heidegger's words that I first read in Giorgio Agamben's *The Open.*

spiritual journey

From my conversations with aAron, a spiritual journey is about awakening, opening, and connecting. This has nothing to do with the dogma from conventional religions. It cannot be dictated by scripture, but must be uncovered through the process of living, which is the process of healing. It is unique to each person. Carl Jung would describe this as an *authentic spiritual journey*. Ram Dass would say this is the reason for incarnation, so a soul can have *human* experiences, to come to Know itself.

all directions are down

This image is a description of the geometry of a black hole, where once you pass the event horizon all directions are down towards the singularity where everything becomes one. It is an image used throughout the book.

Howl

Allen Ginsberg's 1956 poem *Howl* has been one of the most significant artworks in my life. I have listened to several recorded readings where Ginsberg summons the work in different ways: rhythm, timbre, or breath. I was introduced to it eighteen years ago in my English 101 course but never read it. In December 2018 I listened to it and was changed. I felt that Ginsberg had summoned everything he had experienced in a body with a mind and a blistered soul, wailing, howling before Being, expressing his essence, his philosophy of everything in that moment. I also felt moments that I recognized as an artist, moments where he completely dissolved and became a column of air that breathed form from no form. Pure primordial images. This is particularly evident, to me, in the absolute flow of the footnote to Howl, Holy! Holy! Holy!...

Ginsberg's weaving and knotting of physical locations (cities around America), with cosmic time and space, with spiritual locations in visions and hallucinations was a significant source of inspiration for the scales and connections that could be realized in a work of art. The spatiotemporal scales and contradictions that can only really exist in a work of art.

beyond the land

that I saw Charles Stankievech's work *Soniferous Aether of the Land Beyond the Land Beyond* (2013). It is a film shot at the northernmost settlement on Earth—Alert Signals Intelligence Station. The slow-panned time lapses of an Otherworld (not of Earth) attune you to different spatiotemporal scales. It is remarkably visually stunning and a significant contribution to Canadian landscape art. I use this term *beyond the land* throughout the Iqaluit stories.

Death #1

We don't live or die, but float

Referencing Bob Dylan's 1989 song "Man in the Long Black Coat."

gamma-ray burst from another galaxy

These are the most powerful electromagnetic events in the universe, often produced by supernovae during the death of the star and transformation into a neutron star or black hole. It is proposed that the Ordovician-Silurian extinction events from 450 million years ago might have been caused by a gamma-ray burst.

A Dry City

Canada.
When will you be angelic?
When will you take off your clothes?
When will you look at yourself through the grave?

I looked at Canada while I was in Iqaluit, Canada on every street corner. The Canada that decimated the Indigenous Peoples. I looked to my family up north, the trauma, illness, addictions, pain, but also love and laughter. Canada must drop all their stories, guards, clothes and plainly, simply look at themselves through the grave—death—what *we* have done.

Knowing

I do not believe, I Know

A 1959 Interview with Carl Jung on *BBC Four: Face to Face*.

Burkean sublime

Thinking of Edmund Burke's 1757 *A Philosophical Enquiry into the Origin of Our Ideas of the Sublime and Beautiful* as the strongest emotion that the mind is capable of experiencing

// birth | growth | healing | destruction | death | rebirth \\

Becoming-animal

I was first introduced to this concept with Gilles Deleuze and Felix Guattari's *A Thousand Plateaus: Capitalism and Schizophrenia* (1987) in a posthumanities seminar course in my MFA taught by my graduate supervisor, Maria Whiteman. Another reading in this course was Agamben's *The Open*, where the idea of becoming-animal was further developed as he rereads Heidegger. There was a sense that becoming-animal had access to a type of experience that could open to a larger experience with Being. This is also re-emphasized in psychedelic research where returning to a primary state of consciousness, a more primordial form of conscious experience, allows a larger, less constricted reality (see the sections *The Default-Mode Network*, *Entropic Brain*, and *Psilocybin* for more sources, breadcrumbs, notes, and imaginings).

Spending more time with Nietzsche reinforced the notions that becoming does not produce fixed entities or beings, that these are incomplete descriptions of the larger flow of everything.

The idea of *becoming* is continuing to develop in my study of Buddhism and its ontological implications.

An Arts-Based Workshop

Two weeks before leaving for Iqaluit, I was part of the second head and neck cancer image theatre workshop run by David Diamond. It took place in Diane Conrad's arts-based research studio at the University of Alberta. It was a very meaningful event in my life, to return with these wonderful people, and continue to express ourselves. I measured everything against David's movements from that day.

I was two months into my arts-based research class with Diane Conrad in the fall of 2016 when I ran this workshop. Conrad and Beck's (2015) article was a major influence, but there were many readings and activities that influenced this workshop. Below are some of the articles we had read to that point that influenced my disposition to this workshop: Dissanayake's "Art in Global Context: An Evolutionary/Functionalist Perspective for the 21st Century" (2003); Denzin's *Interpretive Ethnography: Ethnographic Practices for the 21st Century* (1997); Ellis, Adams, and Bochner's "Autoethnography: An Overview" (2011); Ermine's "Aboriginal Epistemology" (1995); Spry's "Performing Autoethnography: An Embodied Methodological Praxis" (2001); Boydell's "Making Sense of Collective Events: The Co-creation of a Research-Based Dance" (2011); Springgay, Irwin, and Kind's "A/R/Tographers and Living Inquiry" (2008).

I did not know I was co-creating a work of art. I thought I was just running a workshop. I never knew anyone's name, nor did I foresee the need for image permissions. Everyone agreed to have their photographs taken; otherwise, we would not have restaged them outside. But, because of that missing permission, I have obscured their faces, fittingly, with the healing brush in Photoshop.

The Abyss

Where the doors of perception have been cleansed and everything appears as it is, infinite.

This is a William Blake quote that is the opening quote in Aldous Huxley's *The Doors of Perception.*

whirlpool's event horizon

Lab-generated whirlpools are often used to study event horizons of black holes.

~~You~~

This strikethrough is used throughout the text as an erasure of you, or the self; the unravelling, the emptiness that is unconcealed after becoming nobody, ego-death, awakening, or enlightenment. It is the purest ~~you~~, the ~~you~~ in the open, out in the open ocean, bathing before the abyss. There is a koan in the Zen tradition: *what is your face before even your parents were born?* Something closer to that. Untouched.

radiant jewel, mystical child

Bob Dylan's 1976 "Sara" might have been ringing in my mind.

For Mom, For Dad

This story of a stack of photographs was written in 2012 as part of my MFA and I would read it as I passed water between two claw-footed bathtubs. I exhibited it as a performative film titled *Technique and Time.* In 2015 I performed it live at Rice University, where I sat in the Turrell work of art and the Rothko Chapel. In 2017 I published the story in a collection called *Asylum* published by *Hamilton Arts & Letters.* Brian Webb caught me recycling this old writing in the book and recommend I revisit it with all my life's experiences at my back. On New Year's Eve 2020, then in the morning of the first day in 2021, I put the old text to the side and rewrote it from memory. It barely resembles the original text. It was immensely healing. I love you , Mom / Dad.

And here I am, still dreaming of the sky // you and I always did feel the same

Dreaming of Bob Dylan's 1974 "Tangled Up in Blue," the first song my dad shared of Dylan when I was nineteen.

Lay with life and death hung in the room

With inspiration from Bob Dylan's "I Contain Multitudes" from 2020.

With the sundown, circle moon, comets I relive the past

Bob Dylan's "If You See Her, Say Hello" from 1974.

The Origin of the Work of Art

As noted before, this section was inspired by Martin Heidegger's essay "The Origin of the Work of Art" and Giorgio Agamben's *The Open.* The strife between World and Earth in an artwork as a way to Knowing, to truth, gave me a level of confidence in the transformative potential in art that I only ever saw at the periphery of visions, but now lay in focus at the centre of my mind.

Desert, THE desert

This poem describes the trip and filming that would become *Joshua Tree*, a twenty-five-minute minimalist experimental film I created with Gary James Joynes. It screened in more than ten international film festivals and continues to be exhibited in galleries. It continues to be part of a live dance I am collaborating on with the Brian Webb Dance Company.

Some kind of changing of the guard

Maybe thinking about Bob Dylan's "Changing of the Guards" from 1978.

Visionary Art

Many of aAron and my conversations, no matter the subject—Trump, climate, psilocybin, mediation, art—would always come back to the central idea that all of this was simply the universe expressing itself, for it to come to know itself—a cosmic expression. Knowing through strife, through heaven and hell, bliss and suffering, life and death.

I have seen the term *visionary art* used many times throughout history, but I wanted to carve out a space that was within the vein Carl Jung was writing about in *Modern Man in Search of a Soul.* Thinking about visionary art as a journey towards Individuation, a healing journey, an authentic spiritual journey to the open, that brings our conscious and unconscious worlds in harmony together, revealing themselves to each other. Maybe to self-actualize, liberate, Nirvana. Art as a spiritual practice of healing.

Distant Early Warning

This section draws on Marshall McLuhan's *The McLuhan DEW-Line Newsletter*, which published twenty issues between 1968 and 1970.

E.E. Cummings's 1952 poem "[*i carry your heart with me (i carry it in*]" is how I feel about Candace, it is how I feel about my girls. They are the root of the root that becomes the beautiful tree of life. What I love about the bud of the bud is that a leaf does not come *into* the tree, it comes *out* of the tree, as Alan Watts would say. Just as I did not come *into* this world, but I came *out* of it. It's a nice reorientation. It promises more than it conceals.

The Behaviour of Art

This section is based on Ellen Dissanayake's 1990 *What Is Art For?* A beautiful ethnographic exploration into the behaviour of art and its many functions within human evolution.

Knowing Otherwise

This section is based on Alexis Shotwell's 2011 *Knowing Otherwise*, quote from page 22.

The Default-Mode Network, Entropic Brain, and Psilocybin

Foundational ideas for these sections were inspired by R.L Carhart-Harris et al., "The Entropic Brain" (2014); R. Griffiths et al., "Psilocybin Can Occasion Mystical-Type Experiences" (2006); Timothy Leary et al., *The Psychedelic Experience* (2007); and Michael Pollan, *How to Change Your Mind* (2018). Pollan's excellent book introduced me to the histories, potentials, and futures of psychedelics, while Leary's text is foundational for the understanding of psychedelic ways of knowing.

Along with Paul Stamets's lectures on magic mushrooms, another influential character in my spiritual and psychedelic journey was Terence McKenna who can give spontaneous long-form lectures around perennial philosophies. In one he uses images such as the ocean, abyss, small, large, and medium sizes ideas/stories, and world-transformation. He gave me insights into the nature of consciousness and grounded them in evolutionary psychology. In *Food of the Gods*, he brings these disparate areas of knowledge together in his "Stoned Ape Hypothesis," where he makes the argument that magic mushrooms growing in the scat of tracked prey on the plains of Africa was what triggered the rapid and extreme development of humans' brains and intellect over such a short span of evolutionary time. He is also an exceptional interpreter of Carl Jung. I frequently listen to his recorded lectures, accessible on YouTube.

used for healing and spiritual development in Indigenous Peoples for millennia

I have heard this reference several times in talks but also in Paul Stamets's 1996 guide *Psilocybin Mushrooms of the World: An Identification Guide*. They look at the frequent depiction of mushrooms within ancient cultural artifacts from civilizations that had access to magic mushrooms in their part of the world.

cancer study

Studies on the use of psychedelic drugs and cancer care are growing by the year, and I was initially introduced to this area of research in Pollan's *How to Change Your Mind*, but other initial studies that awakened me to the potential of psilocybin for end-of-life care were S. Ross et al., "Rapid and Sustained Symptom Reduction following Psilocybin Treatment for Anxiety and Depression in Patients with Life-Threatening Cancer" (2016); and C.S. Grob et al., "Pilot Study of Psilocybin Treatment for Anxiety in Patients with Advanced-Stage Cancer" (2011).

they no longer fear death and have learnt how to live

An excellent and beautiful film on fungi as an aware, intelligent, and integral organism in our ecosystems, in which viewers get sustained time with Paul Stamets and his research on fungi, is Louie Schwartzberg's 2019 *Fantastic Fungi*.

In the film, they speak with Dr. Roland Griffiths and two cancer patients. After a psilocybin psychotherapy session, a cancer patient notes,

> In the intense part of this journey, this world and the things that matter to most people, that isn't even what it was about. They say anything mystical can't be explained. It is something like that. It's a feeling of such immense power that you can't even imagine. I have never felt anything like it before. It was about being in a place of infinite space. And just being there...The most glorious part was that it made me feel more comfortable with living, you know, because you're not afraid of dying.

Griffiths, director of Johns Hopkins Center for Psychedelic and Consciousness Research, explains, "There is an experience of positive mood, sometimes open heartedness and love. Transcendence of time and space and then finally it is thought to be ineffable. People say: I can't describe that experience."

Another cancer patient describes their experience:

> In my mind I said, okay, if I give myself over to you, can you promise me that I will be in at least as strong a shape as when I entered this room? And I felt a voice that I needed to heed: *Do you think I would disrespect my own handiwork?* This is the voice from on high: *Do you think I would disrespect my child?* And I felt so beautiful. I felt like I have never felt before. My sense of being loved, of being worthy of love, of being cared for, of being important to someone. It's huge.

openness to experience

D. Erritzoe et al.'s 2019 study "Recreational Use of Psychedelics Is Associated with Elevated Personality Trait Openness" looks at the psychedelic MDMA and finds positive associations between psychedelic experiences and openness to experience. M. Nour et al.'s article "Psychedelics,

Personality and Political Perspectives" (2017) examines the "most intense" psychedelic experiences positively predicting liberal political views, openness and nature relatedness, and negatively predicting authoritarian political views. In a September 29, 2011, news release from Johns Hopkins Medicine, researchers note that their follow-ups fourteen months later still showed lasting changes in the personality trait openness to experience (increased) and may likely be permanent.

significant experience

In *Fantastic Fungi*, Roland Griffiths notes,

> One-third of individuals in the study said it is the single most spiritually significant experience of their lives. About 70 percent say it was among the five most personally meaningful experiences of their lives. And you say, What does that mean? And initially I thought, I wonder if they don't have pretty dull lives? But no, people would say, "You know when my first born came into this world, I'll never forget that and life has never been the same since. Or my father passed away, that was deeply moving to me, I am different now in the world." So you know, it is kind of like that.

meditation reduces DMN activity

In K. Garrison et al.'s 2015 article "Meditation Leads to Reduced Default Mode Network Activity beyond an Active Task," the authors suggest that "meditation leads to relatively reduced default mode processing" (p. 712). In their 2015 article "The Default Mode Network as a Biomarker for Monitoring the Therapeutic Effects of Meditation," R. Simon and M. Engström propose that the DMN could act as "a biomarker for monitoring the therapeutic effects of meditation practices in mental disorders" (p. 1). Lastly, in Taylor et al.'s 2013 article "Impact of Meditation Training on the Default Mode Network during a Restful State," they note,

> Relative to beginners, experienced meditators had weaker functional connectivity between DMN regions involved in self-referential processing and emotional appraisal...These findings suggest that meditation training leads to functional connectivity changes between core DMN regions possibly reflecting strengthened present-moment awareness. (p. 4)

creativity

Arne Dietrich has written several articles since 2000 that have influenced my understandings of the neuroscience and types of creativity. While his initial research focused on discrete regions of the brain, there is much overlap on the connected areas of the Default-Mode Network, which has gained recent focus and study following the publication of many of these articles (Dietrich 2003, 2004a, 2004b, 2019).

In my doctoral dissertation (Necyk, 2019), I describe a mode of creativity put forward by Dietrich called spontaneous-emotional, the closest neuroscience description of a "visionary state" that matches my personal experience:

> *Spontaneous-emotional* creativity, involves the processing of emotional content by emotional-affective structures in the brain which unconsciously processes information that spontaneously pops into consciousness, avoiding the limited attention time and capacity of working memory within the prefrontal cortex. As emotions universally "signify

biologically significant events" (Deitrich, 2004a, p. 1020) creative insights arising into consciousness can engender a phenomenological state akin to a sense of "revelation, an epiphany, or religious experience" (p. 1020), often leading to a strong need for creative expression. Although insights that derive from spontaneous-emotional processing are independent of domain-specific knowledge, Dietrich notes that creative work inspired by such insights "might require specific skills for appropriate expression" (p. 1020)...The prefrontal cortex determines the appropriateness of the insights produced, and is involved in further developing understanding, or integrating "universal," emotional creative insights. (p. 114–15)

The use of the word "universal" immediately resonated with my developing understandings of the collective unconscious from Carl Jung. I see parallels from Carhart-Harris et al.'s 2014 article "The Entropic Brain," where they quote William James's description of the unconscious as

> obviously the larger part of each of us, for it is the abode of everything that is latent and the reservoir of everything that passes unrecorded or unobserved...It is the source of our dreams...In it arise whatever mystical experiences we may have. It is also the fountain-head of much that feeds our religion. In persons deep in religious life—and this is my conclusion—the door into this region seems unusually wide open. (p. 14)

Next they cite Jung:

> The brain is inherited from its ancestors; it is the deposit of the psychic functioning of the whole human race. In the brain, the instincts are preformed, and so are the primordial images which have always been the basis of man's thinking—the whole treasure-house of mythological motifs...Religious symbols have a distinct "revelatory" character; they are usually spontaneous products of unconscious psychic activity...They have developed, plant-like, as natural manifestations of the human psyche. (p. 14)

In my doctoral dissertation, I spent a chapter weaving Deitrich's ideas on the neuroscience of creativity with special emphasis on spontaneous-emotional creativity and universal knowledge, with Carhart-Harris et al.'s entropic brain hypothesis and primary states of consciousness, and Ellen Dissanayake's evolutionarily grounded understanding of the behaviour of art. These were the beginning bridges to understandings around visionary art and how visions, madness, psychedelics, and meditation all knotted together in the DMN.

people living with bipolar or schizophrenia have abnormal DMNs

Through functional MRI scans, D. Öngür et al. (2010) found differences in DMN connectivity between bipolar-control, bipolar-schizophrenia, and schizophrenia-control.

ECT

BLACK COLOUR, NONE NUMBER

Sha once said that this line made him think of depression, so I find myself again aching back to Bob Dylan's 1963 "A Hard Rain's A-Gonna Fall" and Ginsberg's *Howl* (see Ginsberg & Miles, 2006).

A Sermon

Summoning Anne Waldman's poetic reading of shamans during Martin Scorsese's pseudo-documentary *Rolling Thunder Revue: A Bob Dylan Story*.

she erodes the sun; black

Feeling close to Bob Dylan's 1965 "She Belongs to Me."

Music Room

Knotting Ginsberg's *Howl* and *Kaddish* together (see Ginsberg & Miles, 2006; Ginsberg, 2010).

Into Mania

ALL COLOUR, INFINITY

This phrase is in contrast to the description of depression as BLACK COLOUR, NONE NUMBER. Mania and depression are a dipole.

In part IV, I break up the Hawking radiation blackbody spectrum formula and Einstein's general relativity formulas to create a visual poem.

As the poem continues it is written listening to Bob Dylan's 1974 "Shelter from the Storm." There are many images of a ravaged soul finding shelter from the mental storm with a goddess, for me Candace with the priestess image of Luanna.

Now, September 17, 2020

Thinking of Dylan's "Changing of the Guards," "Shelter from the Storm," and "Chimes of Freedom" with Ginsberg's *Kaddish*.

For the young girl next to me, who is still with me

tears of rage

Bob Dylan and Richard Manuel's 1968 song "Tears of Rage" always resonated with me.

The artwork I first wrote about this event was a performative reading called *One Too Many Mornings Part Two*, which was part of my MFA work.

Death #2

This field note records a transcendent experience meditating with the most amazing sunset looking from Victoria towards the mountains of Washington State on July 26, 2020. This was one of the first passages written in the book on August 1, 2020. It was a stream of consciousness where the writing style for the book emerged spontaneously (with prior provocations from Sha). Sha and I went back and forth with the initial passage, mining, developing as much as we could from that original expression. The images that emerged from the vision and the vision-writing are what I went back and built the book around. An origin.

For Candace

Much of the universe's timeline was built from *PBS Space Time* episodes that you can find on YouTube. I have watched these for years, building on the physics I learnt in university during my undergrad. I sketched out as much as I could and filled in some blanks and times with further research.

November 4, 2022, waiting for a delayed ferry to get off island to you, Candace, the centre of my universe. These past three months, we have gone through the unimaginable together. The beginning of your/our healing journey! Each day we breathe: no mud, no lotus. From the richest mud we are growing the most beautiful lotus flower together: happiness, peace, acceptance. I am so grateful each day for the love we create together

> falling // dissolving // white rapids // eroding // vast expanse // the open
> // healing
> I love you, Candace

REFERENCES

Agamben, G. (2004). *The open: Man and animal*. Stanford University Press.

Ahmed, S. (2010). *The promise of happiness.* Duke University Press.

Boydell, K.M. (2011). Making sense of collective events: The co-creation of a research-based dance. *Forum Qualitative Sozialforschung / Forum Qualitative Social Research, 12*(1), Art. 5. http://nbn-resolving.de/urn:nbn:de:0114-fqs110155

Brett-MacLean, P., & McTavish, L. (Eds.). (2019). *Art-medicine collaborative practice: Transforming the experience of head and neck cancer*. University of Alberta Press.

Burke, E. (2017). *A philosophical enquiry into the origin of our ideas of the sublime and beautiful*. University of Notre Dame Press. (Original work published 1757)

Carhart-Harris, R.L., Nutt, D., Leech, R., Hellyer, P.J., Shanahan, M., Feilding, A., Tagliazucchi, E., & Chialvo, D.R. (2014). The entropic brain: A theory of conscious states informed by neuroimaging research with psychedelic drugs. *Frontiers in Human Neuroscience, 8*, https://doi.org/10.3389/fnhum.2014.00020

Chapman, O., & Sawchuk, K. (2012). Research-creation: Intervention, analysis and "family resemblances." *Canadian Journal of Communication, 37*(1), 5–26. https://doi.org/10.22230/cjc.2012v37n1a2489

Conrad, D., & Beck, J. (2015). Toward articulating an arts-based research paradigm: Growing deeper. *UNESCO Observatory Multidisciplinary Journal in the Arts, 5*(1), 1–26.

Dass, R. (1971). *Be here now*. Lama Foundation.

Delany, S.R. (2009). *The jewel-hinged jaw: Notes on the language of science fiction* (Rev. ed.). Wesleyan University Press.

Deleuze, G., & Guattari, F. (1987). *A thousand plateaus: Capitalism and schizophrenia*. (B. Massumi, Trans.). University of Minnesota Press.

Denzin, N.K. (1997). *Interpretive ethnography: Ethnographic practices for the 21st century* Sage.

Dietrich, A. (2003). Functional neuroanatomy of altered states of consciousness: The transient hypofrontality hypothesis. *Consciousness and Cognition, 12*(2), 231–256. https://doi.org/10.1016/S1053-8100(02)00046-6

Dietrich, A. (2004a). The cognitive neuroscience of creativity. *Psychonomic Bulletin & Review, 11*(6), 1011–1026. https://doi.org/10.3758/BF03196731

Dietrich, A. (2004b). Neurocognitive mechanisms underlying the experience of flow. *Consciousness and Cognition, 13*(4), 746–761. https://doi.org/10.1016/j.concog.2004.07.002

Dietrich, A. (2019). Types of creativity. *Psychonomic Bulletin & Review, 26*(1), 1–12. https://doi.org/10.3758/s13423-018-1517-7

Dissanayake, E. (1990). *What is art for?* University of Washington Press.

Dissanayake, E. (2003). Art in global context: An evolutionary/functionalist perspective for the 21st century. *International Journal of Anthropology, 18*(4), 245–258. https://doi.org/10.1007/BF02447909

Dylan, B. (1963). A hard rain's a-gonna fall [Song]. On *The freewheelin' Bob Dylan.* Columbia.

Dylan, B. (1964). Chimes of freedom [Song]. On *Another side of Bob Dylan.* Columbia.

Dylan, B. (1965). She belongs to me [Song]. On *Bringing it all back home.* Columbia.

Dylan, B. (1975). If you see her, say hello [Song]. On *Blood on the tracks.* Columbia.

Dylan, B. (1975). Shelter from the storm [Song]. On *Blood on the tracks.* Columbia.

Dylan, B. (1975). Tangled up in blue [Song]. On *Blood on the tracks.* Columbia.

Dylan, B. (1975). Tears of rage [Song]. On *The basement tapes.* Columbia.

Dylan, B. (1976). Changing of the guards [Song]. On *Street-legal.* Columbia.

Dylan, B. (1976). Sara [Song]. On *Desire.* Columbia.

Dylan, B. (1981). Every grain of sand [Song]. On *Shot of love.* Columbia.

Dylan, B. (1989). Man in the long black coat [Song]. On *Oh Mercy.* Columbia.

Dylan, B. (2009). Beyond here lies nothin' [Song]. On *Together through life.* Columbia.

Dylan, B. (2020). I contain multitudes [Song]. On *Rough and rowdy ways.* Columbia.

Cummings, E.E. (2015). *E.E. Cummings: Complete poems, 1904–1962* (G.J. Firmage, Ed.). Liveright.

Ellis, C., Adams, T.E. & Bochner, A.P. (2011). Autoethnography: An overview. *Forum: Qualitative Social Research, 12*(1). https://doi.org/10.17169/fqs-12.1.1589

Ermine, W. (1995). Aboriginal epistemology. In J. Barman & M. Battiste (Eds.), *First Nations education in Canada: The circle unfolds* (pp. 101–112). UBC Press.

Erritzoe, D., Carhart-Harris, R., Fisher, P.M., Frokjaer, V.G., Knudsen, G.M., & Smith, J. (2019). Recreational use of psychedelics is associated with elevated personality trait openness: Exploration of associations with brain serotonin markers. *Journal of Psychopharmacology, 33*(9), 1068–1075. https://doi.org/10.1177/0269881119827891

Freeman, J. (1959). Interview with Carl Jung [Video]. *BBC Four: Face to face*. Available on YouTube, https://www.youtube.com/watch?v=oBYEFX2dqpM

Garrison, K. A., Zeffiro, T.A., Scheinost, D., Constable, R. T., & Brewer, J.A. (2015). Meditation leads to reduced default mode network activity beyond an active task. *Cognitive, Affective, & Behavioral Neuroscience, 15*(3), 712–720. https://doi.org/10.3758/s13415-015-0358-3

Ginsberg, A., & Miles, B. (2006). *Howl: Original draft facsimile, transcript and variant versions, fully annotated by author, with contemporaneous correspondence, account of first public reading, legal skirmishes, precursor texts and bibliography* (1st Harper Perennial Modern Classics ed.). Harper Perennial Modern Classics. (Original work published 1956.)

Ginsberg, A. (2010). *Kaddish and other poems: 1958–1960* (Expanded 50th anniversary ed.). City Lights Books.

Gould, D. (2009). *Moving politics: Emotion and ACT UP's fight against AIDS*. University of Chicago Press.

Griffiths, R., McCann, U., Richards, W. A., & Jesse, R. (2006). Psilocybin can occasion mystical-type experiences having substantial and sustained personal meaning and spiritual significance. *Psychopharmacology, 187*(3), 268–283. https://doi.org/10.1007/s00213-006-0457-5

Grob, C.S., Chopra, G.S., McKay, C.R., Danforth, A.L., Hagerty, M., Halberstad, A.L., & Greer, G.R. (2011). Pilot study of psilocybin treatment for anxiety in patients with advanced-stage cancer. *Archives of General Psychiatry, 68*(1), 71–78. doi:10.1001/archgenpsychiatry.2010.116

Haddon, R. (2020, May 25). *Calling voices*. Series of Dreams. https://www.seriesofdreams.com/home/2020/5/25/calling-voices

Haraway, D.J. (2003). *The companion species manifesto: Dogs, people, and significant otherness*. Prickly Paradigm Press.

Haraway, D.J. (2015). Anthropocene, Capitalocene, Plantationocene, Chthulucene: Making kin. *Environmental Humanities, 6*(1), 159–165. https://doi.org/10.1215/22011919-3615934

Haraway, D.J. (2016). *Staying with the trouble: Making kin in the Chthulucene*. Duke University Press.

Haraway, D.J. (2016, September). Tentacular thinking: Anthropocene, Capitalocene, Chthulucene. *e-flux, 75*. https://www.e-flux.com/journal/75/67125/tentacular-thinking-anthropocene-capitalocene-chthulucene/

Heidegger, M. (2008). The origin of the work of art. In D. Farrell Krell (Ed.), *Basic Writings*, 1st Harper Perennial Modern Thought Edition (pp. 143–212). HarperCollins. (Original work published 1950)

Heidegger, M., Stambaugh, J., & Schmidt, D.J. (2010). *Being and time* (Rev. ed.). State University of New York Press. (Original work published 1927)

Hoffman, D. (2019). *The case against reality: Why evolution hid the truth from our eyes*. W.W. Norton & Company.

Hoffman, D. (2015, March). *Do we see reality as it is?* [Video]. TED Conferences. https://www.ted.com/talks/donald_hoffman_do_we_see_reality_as_it_is?

Huxley, A. (1959). *The doors of perception; and, Heaven and hell.* Penguin Books.

Institute of Art and Ideas. (2019, September). *The hard problem of consciousness with Donald Hoffman* [Video]. YouTube. https://youtu.be/ZKoowV2i--U

Johns Hopkins Medicine. (2011, September 29). Single dose of hallucinogen may create lasting personality change [News release]. Johns Hopkins University. https://www.hopkinsmedicine.org/news/media/releases/single_dose_of_hallucinogen_may_create_lasting_personality_change

Jung, C.G. (1933). *Modern man in search of a soul*. Harcourt, Brace.

Kajimura, S., Masuda, N., Lau, J.K.L. & Murayama, K. (2020). Focused attention meditation changes the boundary and configuration of functional networks in the brain. *Scientific Reports, 10*(1), 1–11. https://doi.org/10.1038/s41598-020-75396-9

King, T. (2003). *The truth about stories: A Native narrative.* House of Anansi Press.

Leary, T., Metzner, R., Dass, R., & Karma-gli -pa. (2007). *The psychedelic experience: A manual based on the Tibetan book of the dead*. Citadel Press.

Lennon, J., & McCartney, P. (1966). Tomorrow never knows [Song]. On *Revolver.* EMI.

Loveless, N. (2019). *How to make art at the end of the world: A manifesto for research-creation*. Duke University Press.

Mayfield, M.L., Trussell, D. & Ward, P. (Writers), & Ward, P. (Director). (2020, April 20). Annihilation of joy (Season 1, Episode 5) [Netflix episode]. In P. Ward, D. Trussell, A. Canobbio, B. Kalina, & C. Prynoski (Executive Producers), *The midnight gospel*. Oatmeal Maiden; Titmous, Inc.

McKenna, T.K. (1992). *Food of the gods: The search for the original tree of knowledge: A radical history of plants, drugs, and human evolution*. Bantam.

McLuhan, M. (1968–1970). *The McLuhan DEW-Line newsletter*. Human Development Corporation. vol. 1–3. 20 issues.

Miles, B. (2011). *Allen Ginsberg: Beat poet*. Virgin Pub.

Mitchell, J. (1969). Both sides now [Song]. On *Clouds*. Reprise Records.

Morton, T. (2013). *Hyperobjects: Philosophy and ecology after the end of the world*. University of Minnesota Press.

Necyk, B. (2019a). Alberta #3. *The Muse, 9*, 22–28. https://issuu.com/themuse_magazine/docs/the_muse_issue_9

Necyk, B. (2019b). *Telling stories otherwise* [Doctoral dissertation, University of Alberta]. Education & Research Archive. https://doi.org/10.7939/r3-88nk-sr48

Necyk, B., & Harvey, D. (2018). "Like watching a movie": Notes on the possibilities of art in the Anthropocene. In J. Jagodzinski (Ed.), *Interrogating the Anthropocene: Ecology, aesthetics, pedagogy, and the future in question* (pp. 237–251). Palgrave.

Nhât Hạnh, T. (2002). *No death, no fear: Comforting wisdom for life*. Riverhead Press.

Nhât Hạnh, T. (2012). *Love letter to the earth*. Parallax Press.

Nhât Hạnh, T. (2014). *No mud, no lotus: The art of transforming suffering*. Parallax Press.

Nietzsche, F.W. (1989). *Beyond good and evil: Prelude to a philosophy of the future* (W. Kaufmann, Trans.). Vintage Books Edition. (Original work published 1886)

Nour, M., Evans, L., & Carhart-Harris, R. (2017). Psychedelics, personality and political perspectives. *Journal of Psychoactive Drugs, 49*(3), 182–191. https://doi.org/10.1080/02791072.2017.1312643

Öngür, D., Lundy, M., Greenhouse, I., Shinn, A.K., Menon, V., Cohen, B.M., & Renshaw, P.F. (2010). Default mode network abnormalities in bipolar disorder and schizophrenia. *Psychiatry Research: Neuroimaging, 183*(1), 59–68. https://doi.org/10.1016/j.pscychresns.2010.04.008

Ovid. (n.d.). *Tristia*. Ovid (43 BC–17) - Tristia: Book II. Retrieved February 8, 2022, from https://www.poetryintranslation.com/PITBR/Latin/OvidTristiaBkTwo.php#anchor_Toc35314583

PBS Space Time. (2015–2021). *PBS Space Time.* [YouTube channel]. https://www.youtube.com/c/pbsspacetime

Pollan, M. (2018). *How to change your mind: What the new science of psychedelics teaches us about consciousness, dying, addiction, depression, and transcendence*. Penguin Press.

Ross, S., Bossis, A., Guss, J., Malone, T., Mennenga, S.E., Kalliontzi, K., Corby, P., Schmidt, B. L., Su, Z., Cohen, B., Belser, A., Babb, J., & Agin-Liebes, G. (2016). Rapid and sustained symptom reduction following psilocybin treatment for anxiety and depression in patients with life-threatening cancer: A randomized controlled trial. *Journal of Psychopharmacology, 30*(12), 1165–1180. https://doi.org/10.1177/026988111667551

Schwartzberg, L. (Director). (2019). *Fantastic fungi* [Film]. Moving Art.

Scorsese, M. (Director). (2019). *Rolling thunder revue: A Bob Dylan story by Martin Scorsese.* [Netflix video]. Grey Water Park Productions; Sikelia Productions.

Scorsese, M. (Director), & Rosen, J., Tedeschi, D., Dylan, B., Baez, J., Ginsberg, A., Seeger, P., Muldaur, M., Clancy, L., & Staples, M. (Performers). (2005). *No direction home: Bob Dylan* [Film]. Paramount.

Shotwell, A. (2011). *Knowing otherwise: Race, gender, and implicit understanding.* Penn State University Press.

Simon, R., & Engström, M. (2015). The default mode network as a biomarker for monitoring the therapeutic effects of meditation. *Frontiers in Psychology, 6.* https://doi.org/10.3389/fpsyg.2015.00776

Sinner, A., & Conrad, D. (Eds.). (2015). *Creating together: Participatory, community-based, and collaborative arts practices and scholarship across Canada*. Wilfrid Laurier University Press.

Sontag, S. (1979). *Illness as metaphor* (1st Vintage Books edition.). Vintage Books.

Springgay, S., Irwin, R.L. & Kind, S. (2008). A/R/Tographers and living inquiry. In G. Knowles & A. Cole (Eds.), *Handbook of the arts in qualitative research* (pp. 83–93). Sage.

Spry, T. (2001). Performing autoethnography: An embodied methodological praxis. *Qualitative Inquiry, 7*(6), 706–732.

Stamets, P. (1996). *Psilocybin mushrooms of the world: An identification guide*. Ten Speed Press.

Stankievech, C. (2013). *The soniferous aether of the land beyond the land beyond* [35 mm film]. Montreal Museum of Fine Arts. https://www.mbam.qc.ca/en/works/67249/

Suzuki, S., & Dixon, T. (1982). *Zen mind, beginner's mind*. Weatherhill.

Taylor, V.A., Daneault, V., Grant, J., Scavone, G., Breton, E., Roffe-Vidal, S., Courtemanche, J., Lavarenne, A. S., Marrelec, G., Benali, H., & Beauregard, M. (2013). Impact of meditation training on the default mode network during a restful state. *Social Cognitive & Affective Neuroscience, 8*(1), 4–14. https://doi.org/10.1093/scan/nsr087

Thomas, R.F. (2017). *Why Bob Dylan matters*. William Collins.

Tzu, L. (2021). *Tao te ching: Power for the peaceful* (M. Mullinax, Trans.). Fortress Press.

Unitarian Universalist Association. (n.d.). *Indra's magnificent jeweled net*. https://www.uua.org/re/tapestry/youth/bridges/workshop7/indra

Von Uexküll, J. (2010). *A foray into the worlds of animals and humans: With a theory of meaning*. University of Minnesota Press.

Watts, A. (1957). *Way of zen.* Pantheon.

Watts, A. (n.d.). *Ecological awareness*. The Library of Consciousness. https://www.organism.earth/library/document/ecological-awareness

Watts, A., & Huang, A.C. (1975). *Tao: The watercourse way*. Pantheon Books.

Weiner, E. (2012, March 9). Where heaven and earth come closer. *The New York Times,* 10. https://www.nytimes.com/2012/03/11/travel/thin-places-where-we-are-jolted-out-of-old-ways-of-seeing-the-world.html